Teaching Reading Sourcebook 2022-2023

Gota Idan

Educating AND LEARNING

Advanced education

Understudy learning in advanced education is an element of both formal and casual encounters. Formal learning happens because of a homeroom or related action organized by an instructor as well as others to assist understudies with accomplishing indicated mental, or other, goals. Casual learning envelops the wide range of various results of understudies' support in an advanced education experience. In the two cases, the more expanded or complete the experience, the more prominent the possible impact. In a thorough 1991 review, Ernest Pasquarelli and Patrick Terenzini depicted the manners by which school influences understudies as for some sorts of learning. While they found that proper learning connected with scholarly and mental abilities, and to topic skill, casual learning was displayed to influence on numerous different regions.

Confusions emerge, in any case, in light of the number and assortment of factors influencing school learning. For instance, while the distinctions between being a private understudy and a suburbanite understudy don't appear to enormously influence mental or topic learning, they are generally persuasive regarding psychosocial change, scholarly and social qualities, freedom, and comparative variables. Is this absolutely a nearby versus off-grounds distinction? Age might be a mediating variable in such cases, since one would anticipate more seasoned, working grown-ups (a continually developing understudy populace in all of advanced education) to address a significant level of understudies living off-grounds. Considering that less psychosocial change may be normal with such students in light of the fact that their mentalities and values are now deep rooted the noticed contrasts among on-and off-grounds learning could be a component of understudy segment contrasts like age, as well as the actual climate. For instance, while the impact of school on the scholarly and social upsides of occupant understudies is huge, this impact determines a lot of its effect from drenching in the school climate and the development of more youthful students who may nothave had a wide scope of involvement. Grown-up, non-inhabitant students might have all the more prized convictions and a more extensive scope of involvement and by straightforward development, may as of now have grown more refined sets of values. Subsequently not just area has the effect, yet the blend of area and attributes of the students.

The Theory behind the Practice

At the point when the main version of this reference book was distributed in 1971, the overarching way to deal with educating and learning was the behaviorist model. Created by B. F. Skinner and others during the 1950s, this model thought about boosts like informative occasions or exercises, the reactions of students to these upgrades, and possibilities or results in light of those reactions. The essential recommendation was that learning happened when the ideal reactions were inspired by the boosts. Robert Manger's work with educational targets (exact explanations of planned ways of behaving alongside estimation measures) and Benjamin Bloom and associate's 1956 scientific categorizations (characterization plans) of goals were additionally significant effects on the manners by which guidance was designed and conveyed. The ordered levels are information, perception, application, examination, combination, and assessment. A down to earth issue for instructors is that there can be goals for in a real sense each educational movement and each sort of conduct from securing fundamental information to study hall mindfulness and the improvement of significant worth frameworks. While behaviorism has been to a great extent supplanted as an informative hypothesis, the fundamental worth of clear targets, proper estimation measures, and the particular of different sorts of wanted learning have stayed as significant rudiments for planning powerful guidance.

Mental hypothesis, basically the place that learning includes the student's relationship of new upgrades with existing ideas and order plans, recovered some help during the 1970s and has kept on creating in its applications since that time. Marilla Svinicki (1999) framed five general procedures for instructing that get from the early hypothesis: (1) coordinating understudies' consideration through verbal or viewable signals; (2) stressing how material is coordinated, again with different prompts; (3) making data more significant by furnishing relationship with other material or applications; (4) empowering dynamic checking of grasping through addressing and criticism; and (5) making up for cutoff points of data handling and memory frameworks with more modest measures of data, survey, breaks, and centering consideration.

Metacognition, or contemplating thinking, went past straightforward affiliations and brought students more into the course of effectively maneuvering new data and consolidating it toward both their own applied plans and those of the subject in question. Svinicki proposes that educators ought to show and portray their own reasoning as they deal with through issues, stress critical thinking and other exercises that give valuable chances to rehearsing points of view, and even show explicit systems when important. The educator, as the master in a particular field, turns into a mental coach and uses such strategies to assist understudies with moving from positions as tenderfoots in the discipline to additional carefully prepared specialists. Instructors in this manner furnish understudies with devices for understanding and managing future, more mind boggling material. Since effective critical thinking methodologies improve execution, the extra advantage is persuasive: it expands understudies' assumptions for fruitful culmination of the work and reinforces their convictions about their capacity to accomplish the work.

Student focused guidance is a term that alludes to taking care of a student's singular requirements, contrasts, and capacities, as well as to sharing liability regarding learning. Research by Paul Pint rich (1995) has laid out that understudies who can handle their own way of behaving, inspiration, and comprehension are by and large fruitful in school. Such understudies self-manage their learning in three ways. In the first place, they practice dynamic control by checking what they do, why they make it happen, and what occurs and afterward adapting. Second, they have objectives that mark wanted execution levels and they utilize these while choosing what changes in accordance with make. Third, they acknowledge that the control should be theirs as opposed to another person's. These methodologies rotate around the significant basic idea that students can practice control and impact instructive results, and that doing so has many advantages.

Cooperative learning is the act of effectively captivating students in joint disclosure, examination, and utilization of data. It has its foundations in the force of companion and different gatherings to impact the advancement of understandings, values, and convictions. According to a realistic point of view, cooperative learning is likewise a more delegate model of contemporary practice in the functioning scene. In a fascinating incongruity, notwithstanding, understudies who have been by and large fruitful in educator focused models tend, from the beginning, to dismiss cooperative advancing as a relinquishment of the instructor's liability, accepting that the occupation of conveying content has been moved to different understudies. This is an error of the reason for cooperation, and it represents an unexpected issue for educators: arranging and organizing cooperative work so that students' jobs and responsibilities are clear, and furthermore making it evident that the instructor is serving unique, however similarly significant jobs as an asset, an aide, a guide, an assessor, and any of a few different jobs. Understudies are not supposed to show one another; they are supposed to cooperate to arrive at suitable objectives. The worth of self-managed learning is clear in this specific situation. All around developed cooperative work recognizes student obligations, lays out objectives, gives students chances to think about the objectives and to structure their own endeavors in like manner, and supports helpful exertion. Svinicki proposes the accompanying techniques for advancing student focused guidance: (1) energize self-guideline; (2) utilize cooperative techniques; (3) utilize critical thinking exercises that interface content to genuine circumstances; and (4) give models of the cycles, methodologies, and propensities for thought about the discipline being educated.

Educating and Its Outcomes

There isn't adequate room here to give subtleties of the multitude of connections between different sorts of learning and educating procedures. More complete portrayals are accessible in Kenneth Feldman and Michael Paulsen's 1998 conversation of school showing and learning and in How College Affects Students (1991) by Pasquarelli and Terenzini. A few essential discoveries from that work are separated and framed beneath, and the association of the accompanying passages follows that of the sections in Pasquarelli and Terenzini's message.

For verbal, quantitative, and topic getting the hang of, addressing gives off an impression of being a significant strategy, especially in learning material at the information and understanding levels of the Bloom et al. scientific categorization. Individualized guidance in different structures appears to be sensibly viable in showing comparative substance. More complex mental targets and emotional goals show up better realized whenever open doors for connection happen, as in more modest classes and those that utilization conversation and dynamic learning strategies. Cooperative advancing likewise furnishes students with various elective clarifications that should be accommodated, and endeavors toward this path support accomplishment of both complex mental and emotional goals for learning content material.

At the point when general mental abilities and scholarly development are wanted, a cycle including investigation of data, creating clarifications, and it is valuable to arrive at speculations. Like the experiential model of David Kolb (1984), this cycle is reiterative, and its solidarity is in the requirement for students to go past retention of realities and into tackling issues through finding relevant information, testing potential speculations, and coming to end results. The mental practice associated with such exercises gives valuable preparation that can be moved. Furthermore, the need to examine and discuss the benefits of clashing contentions gives potential chances to foster composed and spoken relational abilities. Comparative strategies support scholarly development, decisive reasoning, and the capacity to manage thoughtfully complex issues. Nonetheless, a solitary course experience may not deliver huge outcomes; additional time and openness are for the most part essential.

The psychosocial changes portrayed by Pasquarelli and Terenzini incorporate inner matters like personality and confidence, as well as outer factors like associations with individuals and builds in the rest of the world. In the inside psychosocial domain, there don't appear to be many impacts that can be straightforwardly ascribed to school educating and learning, or even to the general school climate. One explanation presented by Pasquarelli and Terenzini for the absence of huge or significant discoveries is the trouble in estimating such changes. Research misses the mark on commonly acknowledged set of speculations to direct the work, and estimation itself is loose. They likewise note the range of college environments and the trouble in summing up from information accumulated across these conditions. Another explanation might be that going to school doesn't ensure a continuously sure arrangement of encounters. Scholarly challenges can affect confidence, and examination proposes that numerous understudies leave school in light of a feeling of segregation and dejection. Such adverse results can offset the constructive outcomes of school, subsequently reducing the general strength of the discoveries.

There are things that should be possible to keep away from such issues. Arthur Checkering and Zelda Gammon (1987) fostered a rundown of "Seven Principles for Good Practice in Undergraduate Education." They propose that guidance that supports social and scholastic connection, helpful endeavors, dynamic learning, ordinary criticism, exclusive standards about both understudy exertion and results, and the production of regard and trust among people and gatherings are basic to progress.

As far as changes concerning outside factors, Pasquarelli and Terenzini report general understudy acquires in autonomy, no authoritarian thinking, tolerance, scholarly direction, development, individual change abilities, and self-awareness. That's what they note "the biggest first year recruit senior changes seem, by all accounts, to be away from tyrant, stubborn, and ethnocentric reasoning and conduct" (p. 257).

Educators can do a lot to help the sorts of development that have been found in the outside psychosocial region. The utilization of helpful and cooperative techniques for instructing and learning upholds the improvement of interactive abilities and group enrollment abilities, and furthermore opens understudies to various sentiments and thoughts. Educators can introduce assorted perspectives and draw in understudies in investigation, examination, and blend of these perspectives. To be sure, most guidance that tends to the upper levels of the Bloom scientific classification (i.e., examination, union, and assessment) expects understudies to gauge the benefits of elective thoughts and approaches, and to make proof based decisions. As understudies move from section level courses through graduation and into graduate instruction, there is an undeniably weighty weight on autonomous learning and the improvement of the capacity to complete one's own investigations and come to one's own end results. It isnot astounding then, that one of the most mind-blowing recorded impacts of school is an expansion in the internality of understudies' locus of control. Locus is one part of attribution hypothesis, and it alludes to the understudy's view of the degree to which she or he has the ability to impact results. Those understudies whose locus is more inner (the people who are for the most part effective) feel fit for practicing a control and they make a move to do as such, while understudies who show outer inclinations are by and large less fruitful and have not many sensations of force or the capacity to influence results. They are much of the time more aloof and characteristic their disappointments (and once in a while, even their triumphs) to outer factors such the expertise of the educator, their schoolmates, course trouble or straightforwardness, and even, to karma.

Likewise, with outer psychosocial factors, various perspectives and values appear to change in school, and there appears to be a sensible connection between these sorts of changes as far as their tendency as well as in the sorts of guidance that can advance development. Attitudinal changes happen in social, stylish, and scholarly regions and are set apart by more noteworthy refinement and interest in more extensive scopes of music, writing, reasoning, imaginative exercises, history, and the humanities. Different changes are tracked down in instructive and word related values, remembering such things as interest for liberal training and the longing for a satisfying profession. More change appears to happen in the early long stretches of school than does in the last years. Projects and organizations that help (especially) more youthful students all along and that consolidate sound educational techniques, the improvement of a feeling of commitment in a scholarly local area, and promptly accessible help administrations set out many open doors for progress.

To the extent that ethical advancement is concerned, going to school appears to advance development toward principled moral thinking reliably. This development happens essentially in the early long periods of school and it is reflected in both in-school and post-graduation conduct. Pasquarelli and Terenzini report this change as one of the most unmistakable, yet they likewise note that proof of progress doesn't tell how or why such change happens. There are a few legitimate associations with showing methodologies around here, and they are like those prominent above. For instance, utilization of the conversation strategy, cooperative learning, peer audit, and different procedures that expect understudies to think about elective perspectives and to accommodate contrasts among these other options, can prompt more receptiveness to novel thoughts, more social responsiveness, and more consciousness of social/moral issues. Such procedures can be utilized in many teaches and are not restricted to specific courses managing moral thinking, morals, and related subjects. In these or different courses, presenting understudies to certifiable moral issues and expecting them to propose elective answers for issues utilizing the viewpoints of the different partners is one method for exhibiting the intricacies of settling on such choices. Such a methodology can likewise assist with extending the understudies' scope of comprehension of contrasting perspectives.

One of the benefits of advanced education's accentuation on variety and multicultural issues is that the scope of encounters and assessments accessible for discussion is impressively widened. This benefit connects with research discoveries that ethical thinking doesn't create so a lot, or as reliably, in settings where there is a serious level of comparability among understudies. Homogeneity will in general lessen the clashing sentiments that are the reason for conversation and blend.

The Importance of Individual Differences and Motivation

In spite of a lot of conversation and the improvement of an enormous number of blueprint and marks of individual distinction, some watchfulness is important while thinking about their belongings. Individual contrasts like general insight, partiality for specific subjects, level of information, earlier preparation, individual experience, and social and related contrasts can be recognized sensibly well and considered. Different factors, be that as it may, are not so much saw but rather more hard to accommodate when guidance is planned. One area of discussion is over that gathering of contrasts known as educating and learning styles.

While it is for the most part concurred that every individual might have a few remarkable blends of qualities, and that sure of these qualities can be distinguished and sorted, making oversimplified presumptions about style is hazardous. For sure, there are such countless various characterizations of style and individual contrast, that it is quite simple to expect one-sided dependence on any one, or to endeavor to incorporate too much. Research recommends that since most students have a collection of styles, essentially utilizing various informative techniques will give the larger part adequate chances to learn. While understudies might utilize a few methodologies more as often as possible than others, they can adjust to new circumstances by utilizing anything elective methodologies appear to be generally reasonable right now. Those couple of students have restricted collections who have the best trouble and for whom the best facilities are important. Valuable mediations for these students incorporate individual help, making guidance more concrete and pertinent through relating content to genuine circumstances or to their own encounters, making sense of cycles for arranging content data, showing general review abilities as well as unambiguous critical thinking methodologies, utilizing continuous appraisal strategies, and giving standard input.

Inspiration is a well-informed region, and however there are a few depictions of the components of inspiration, these components are very comparable. Michael Thrall's 1998 refining of thirteen persuasive methodologies brought about a six-thing conceptualization that applies to advanced education understudies and personnel. The components were: consideration, mentality, meaning, skill, authority, and fulfillment. Of the models explored, one that can be straightforwardly associated with school instructing is that of John Keller (1983). Keller proposed a model for the persuasive plan of guidance. The model layouts a pattern of data sources, occasions, and outcomes that could bring about sure or adverse results. Understudies and educators go into an instructing learning circumstance with sets of values and assumptions that influence the degree and nature of the work they use. Uplifting perspectives (e.g., the understudy is keen regarding the matter; the educator has done explore on the point) and assumptions (e.g., the understudies trust themselves to be capable in the substance region; the educator anticipates that the course should be generally welcomed) lead to more prominent exertion, and exertion straightforwardly influences execution. Solid execution prompts both fulfillment (through the outcomes of passing marks, the feeling of a "wonderful piece of handiwork" and the acknowledgment of viable learning) and elevated value and assumptions for the future (which further inspire exertion). In any case, in the negative heading, certain mentalities (e.g., the understudies would rather not take the class; the educator is worn out on showing the material) and assumptions (e.g., an understudy's subject tension; the educator's interests about the course) can lessen exertion and lead to decreased execution and disillusionment, subsequently building up bad perspectives and assumptions.

Raymond Wlodkowski (1998) stresses that inborn inspiration is all the more remarkable that outward inspiration. At the end of the day, the more seasoned perspective on inspiration as something done to somebody is less pertinent than the comprehension that achievement includes advancing or making sets of conditions under which the individual is the person who really gives the inspiration. A normal case in school learning would be an educator's making of sets of encounters that stimulate the understudies' advantage and permit commitment in exercises that both advance development and give potential open doors to progress. In this situation, fulfillment comes inside from achievement, while grades are just a documentation of the learning and fulfillment, as opposed to sometime later rewards that drive execution.

Deciding Outcomes

The development of both assessment and appraisal has been outstanding, and with this development have come assumptions that educators and organizations will actually want to archive their presentation, and that of their understudies, in significant ways.

Study hall tests are presently not adequate as proof. Affirmation and licensure are significant in specific expert fields, however many disciplines don't need such normalized exhibitions of learning, and many have addressed even these all the more painstakingly built measures as far as their capacity to portray advancing genuinely.

Besides, the interest of certifying bodies isn't just in that frame of mind of information are gathered in what ways, yet additionally in what moves have been made because of appraisals. As such, evaluation has turned into a cycle for ceaseless correction and improvement. Appraisal is worried about the aftereffects of instructing and the instructive experience, and of deciding as definitively as conceivable what was realized. This job contrasts from that of assessment, which is more a cycle to decide legitimacy or worth. Assessment is a more worldwide, formal, quantitative, and intermittent interaction, while evaluation is in many cases tighter, casual, subjective, and progressing. This is on the grounds that evaluation's goals are frequently at the level of the singular student and less manageable to sociology research strategies that rely upon tests of sufficient size to permit factual induction. Strangely, both assessment and evaluation utilize the terms formative, meaning a cycle for investigation, modification, and improvement; and summative, meaning an interaction for deciding legitimacy and coming to managerial conclusions about individuals or projects.

The most broadly circled and complete wellspring of evaluation data is Classroom Assessment Techniques (1993) by Thomas Angelo and K. Patricia Cross. This book contains various strategies for evaluating learning in the quick setting of the homeroom, as well as in the more extensive setting of the full course, the school semester, and then some. During the 1990s, this work and the simultaneous interest in Ernest Boyer's origination of the grant of instructing prompted the advancement of strategies for study hall research that are, as per Cross and Mimi Steadman (1996), student focused, educator coordinated, cooperative, setting explicit, academic, pragmatic/applicable, and nonstop. Especially like evaluation in its accentuation on learning, study hall research gave an extension that associated examination of homeroom learning with the more conventional exploration that had recently held elite freedoms to the term grant. As a result, assessment and evaluation techniques were mixed to give a vehicle for the educator researcher to do the grant of instructing.

Grown-up Learning and the Growth of Technology

A new and one of a kind situation emerged during the 1990s because of the expansion in the quantity of grown-up students and projects open a good way off. Not exclusively was this populace of understudies totally different from conventional, private understudies, however the settings of instructing and learning were additionally extraordinarily unique.

Stephen Brookfield (1991) recommends six standards for successfully working with grown-up learners:(1) willful investment and commitment by students; (2) regard among members and affirmation of students' encounters and information; (3) cooperative instead of mandate help of students' encounters; (4) praxis and consistent coordination of exercises into a brought together entire; (5) basic reflection; and (6) advancing personally managed endeavors and a feeling of strengthening. In any case, since most of grown-up students are suburbanites or understudies removing courses from the conventional grounds setting, the advantages of the customary networks of the school grounds are not promptly accessible to this populace, and potential open doors for casual exchange, for creating social relationships, and for investing gathered energy in course prerequisites are restricted.

While these issues about new understudy populaces were being examined, the quick development of distance schooling programs, particularly courses and educational plans conveyed totally, or primarily, by means of the Internet, was bringing up issues about how guidance could be conveyed in an immaterial structure. Rena Pall off and Keith Pratt (2001) recommend that the accompanying illustrations have been advanced up to this point: (1) course improvement necessities to zero in on intuitiveness, not content, since regardless of whether course satisfied is known and laid out, there stays the need to convey it in manners that work with learning; (2) personnel and understudy jobs need to change, with less accentuation on uneven conveyance and more on dynamic and intuitive modes; (3) staff and understudy preparing on the utilization of the innovation, as well as the new methods of guidance, is basic to progress; (4) workforce and understudies need to have significant encouraging groups of people all through the course insight; (5) establishments should foster masterful plans that work out in a good way past mechanical prerequisites and manage everything from pedagogical support to protected innovation freedoms; (6) foundations probably tried and solid framework set up, and the frameworks utilized ought to be open and usable; (7) advances ought to be picked by groups of clients, and decisions ought to be situated in educational as well as specialized boundaries.

Outline

Starting around 1970 there have been many changes in advanced education changes that middle on various understudy populaces, various strategies for conveying guidance, and various originations of what an advanced degree is and the way in which it ought to be sought after. This change cycle will proceed, yet regardless of desperate expectations that innovation will swap the requirement for school grounds, almost certainly, the private experience of undergrad instruction and the escalated idea of graduate preparation will keep on requiring amazing open doors for connection and apprenticeship that must be given on conventional grounds.

Worldwide PERSPECTIVE

An inquisitive conundrum should be visible as one thinks about tutoring and showing across the many societies of the world. From one perspective there is huge variety among societies and inside most societies in the ways in which individuals learn.

Simultaneously there is a momentous closeness across countries in the ways where chances to learn are given through conventional schools and educational systems.

Anthropologists, and teachers who have shown in various social settings, have long noted contrasts in the ways that youngsters naturally introduced to various social settings figure out how to learn. While there are varieties inside any social gathering some of the time across a tight scope of distinction, and some of the time across a wide reach (such contrasts are regularly alluded to as individual learning styles)- obviously discernible modular contrasts among social gatherings have been indisputable. Such contrasts are breaking down in the writing of European pioneer states, like the United States, Canada, Australia, and New Zealand, which contain references to contrasts in ways to deal with, and understanding of, learning between the European pilgrim/colonizer gatherings and the first native occupants, and among pilgrims and all the more as of late shown up worker bunches from region of the world other than Europe. These distinctions have additionally figured unmistakably in examinations of schooling in other provincial and postcolonial (or neocolonial) states all over the planet. However, with a rising consciousness of these impressive varieties in realizing, there has at the same time spread all through the world a standard model of tutoring, which frequently doesn't consider these distinctions, and subsequently frequently causes extensive harm to the learning capability of youngsters.

It is habitually failed to remember that tutoring, as it has come to be known, is only one of a huge range of social foundations that people have imagined to give valuable open doors to youngsters to learn. It is, truth be told, a human development of moderately late beginning, on a mass scale. The expansive scope arrangement of training as an instrument of statecraft and state improvement was really "imagined" in Prussia later, and because of, the Napoleonic attack of that country. It spread rapidly all through Europe and other generally affluent nations of the time, and all the more slowly across the world through frontier burden and, now and again, through social acquiring. Be that as it may, in the wide scope of history it is a very new friendly establishment. In its crucial structures (thus the term formal schooling) it was set by the experience, perspectives, and comprehension of the mid-to late-nineteenth century elites in the then recently industrialized countries. As those essential structures have spread all over the planet they have scarcely changed, even in the richest countries, for well more than hundred years. That standard model for the most part includes, all over the planet, the accompanying fundamental components.

One hundred to a few hundred kids/youth gathered (frequently necessarily for a time of years) in a structure called a school, from roughly the age of six or seven up to somewhere close to mature eleven and sixteen.

Guidance goes on for three to six hours out of each day, five or six days of the week.

Understudies are isolated into gatherings of twenty to sixty people.

Understudies work with a solitary grown-up (a "confirmed" educator) in a solitary space for (particularly in the upper grades) discrete times of forty to sixty minutes, each gave to a different subject.

Subjects are considered and educated in a gathering of youngsters of generally a similar age, with supporting learning materials, like books, blackboards, note pads, exercise manuals and worksheets, and, progressively, PCs (and in specialized regions such things as research facilities, workbenches, and practice destinations).

There is a standard educational program, set by a power level a lot of over the singular school (regularly a focal or commonplace/state government), and which all understudies are supposed to cover during a time reviewed style.

Grown-ups, thought to be more proficient, educate, and understudies get guidance from them.

Assuming they are to go any higher in the tutoring framework, understudies are supposed and expected to echo once again to the grown-ups what they have been educated.

Educators or potentially a focal assessment framework assess understudies' capacity to echo once again to them what the understudies have been instructed, and furthermore give formal perceived certifications to passing specific grades or levels.

Most or all of the monetary help comes from public or regional governments, or different sorts of power places (for example church-related schools) well over the nearby local area level.

There are various clarifications or speculations in regards to how and why this specific example of arranging and giving educating to youngsters has become generally overlaid upon the wide variety of manners by which youngsters figure out how to learn. Inside this cross-public conundrum, there is incongruity. While it has been plainly exhibited that this standard model of instructing and tutoring has habitually demonstrated extremely useless for gaining among youngsters from social gatherings not quite the same as its place of beginning, the amassed writing from mental and learning brain science, human studies, and similar training has progressively shown that it is likewise intrinsically broken for kids (and grown-ups besides) from those very societies of beginning.

The framework, so, is innately wasteful and insufficient. Individuals of each and every age and culture just don't learn well under these game plans.

These conventional, yet presently almost general, examples of instructing and tutoring are a curio of the misguided judgments of an alternate time and, for a significant part of the world, a better place. In any case, now that examples are set up, it appears to be almost difficult to dispose of them, and, surprisingly, the most extravagant countries can adjust them just marginally at extraordinary exertion and cost, and normally just over extremely extensive stretches of time.

In the end many years of the 20th hundred years, in any case, another example started to show up in agricultural countries where the European framework has demonstrated to be so frequently broken for learning. Educational systems have started to give the idea that are breaking the types of formal tutoring in very major ways, and that are delivering striking learning gains among very poor and underestimated youngsters. Starting around 2002 more than 100 of these instructing/school programs have been recorded, some including tens or many schools, others a huge number of schools. A few normal elements of these elective types of tutoring are these:

Youngster focused instead of instructor driven teaching method

Dynamic instead of inactive learning

Multigraded study halls with persistent advancement learning

Peer-mentoring more established or potentially quicker learning kids help and "educate" more youthful as well as more slow learning youngsters

Painstakingly created independent learning materials, which youngsters, alone or in little gatherings, can manage themselves, at their own speed, with assistance from different understudies and educators as fundamental the kids are answerable for their own learning

Mixes of completely prepared educators, to some degree prepared educators, and local area asset human guardians and other local area individuals are vigorously associated with the learning of the youngsters, and in the administration of the school

Dynamic understudy contribution in the administration and the executives of the school

Free progressions of youngsters and grown-ups between the school and the local area

Local area association incorporates thoughtfulness regarding the nourishment and wellbeing needs of small kids some time before they arrive at young

Privately adjusted changes in the pattern of the school day or the school year

Continuous observing/assessment/criticism frameworks permitting the "framework" to gain from its own insight, with consistent change of/trial and error with the approach

Progressing and exceptionally successive in-administration educator advancement programs, with weighty utilization of friend tutoring

Early signs recommend that they are undeniably more adaptable and effective in adjusting their educating/tutoring ways to deal with the varieties among societies in how individuals figure out how to learn. In any case, minimal serious exploration has been finished to attempt to comprehend how and why these new projects appear to function admirably in advancing learning among extremely assorted gatherings. That is quite difficult for the twenty-first 100 years.

Information BASES OF

Analysts and different researchers trying to comprehend and characterize the information and thinking basic instructing have zeroed in on various issues and present numerous points of view as a powerful influence for this perplexing space. Quite a bit of this work has tended to a blend of three arrangements of interrelated questions:

What do (or ought to) educators know? What spaces or classes of information are significant for educating?

How do instructors be aware? What is the nature or type of different sorts of information required for educating?

Do educators' think process? Thought process processes underlie educating?

Endeavors to resolve these inquiries are persuaded, to some extent, by the association between how educators instruct and educators' thought process, know, and accept.

Authentic Overview

During the principal half of the 20th century the substance and nature of educators' information was generally unproblematic. In light of different appraisals for educator certificate of the period, instructors had to realize the substance that they would show understudies and have some information on educational practice. As precise projects of examination on instructing started to arise during the 1960s, consideration moved to different instructor qualities and ways of behaving related with expanded understudy accomplishment. In spite of the fact that this research didn't straightforwardly inspect the information or considering educators, it was grounded in a presumption that information on connections laid out through deliberate examination could give a "logical reason for the craft of instructing," as the title of the 1978 book by Nathaniel L. Gage proposed.

As brain research moved from conduct to mental points of view, researchers of showing stuck to this same pattern and started to zero in on the psychological existence of educators. By the 1980s, mental analysts had laid out that the aggregation of rich assemblages of information is basic to master execution in different areas, going from chess playing to clinical analysis. Researchers of instructing started attempting to describe the master information that is required for good educating. In 1986 Lee S. Shulman catalyzed interest in the methodical investigation of the information fundamental educating, contending particularly for the significance of understanding the job of educators' information on the substance they instruct.

Spaces of Knowledge for Teaching

Instructing is a complicated demonstration, requiring numerous sorts of information. Some of this knowledge is general and genuinely getting through like information on topic content or of general educational standards; some is more unambiguous and transient, for example, information on the specific understudies being instructed and what has occurred in a specific class. Different frameworks for portraying the information required for instructing have been created with changing accentuations and purposes. With any arrangement of classes or spaces of information, it is vital to remember that these frameworks are accustomed to carry applied request to information that is in all actuality perplexing and interrelated. The different classifications of information are not discrete elements, and the limits between spaces are fluffy, best case scenario. In light of these provisos, the accompanying arrangement of classes of educator information is approximately founded on a 1987 article by Shulman:

Information on topic content

Information on broad educational standards and techniques

Information on students, their qualities, and how they learn

Information on instructive settings

Information on instructive objectives, purposes, and values

Since they are vital to the everyday work of educators, general academic information, information about students, and information on topic have been the focal point of extensive exploration and insightful talk.

General instructive information/information about students. These firmly related classifications of educator information incorporate information about instructing, learning, and students that isn't well defined for the educating of specific topic content. One huge part of this area is information on homeroom the board information on the most proficient method to keep gatherings of understudies drew in with different study hall errands. Instructors should have collections of schedules and techniques for laying out homeroom strategies, arranging homeroom occasions, keeping exercises on target, and responding to understudy misconduct. Instructors likewise endless supply of educational procedures for orchestrating homeroom conditions and directing illustrations to advance understudy learning. Experienced educators have collections of methodologies and schedules for leading illustrations, keeping them moving along as planned, and advancing understudy commitment.

Educators' information about overseeing study halls and directing illustrations is interwoven with information and convictions about students, learning, and instructing. Hypotheses about how understudies learn guide educators' educational choices and collaborations with understudies, frequently in an understood way. For instance, an educator who imagines the student's job as a latent beneficiary of information instructs uniquely in contrast to one who considers the student's job as a functioning member in the growing experience. The previous commonly presents data that understudies are supposed to take care of, trailed by practice and practice of the introduced data. The last option is able to introduce critical thinking circumstances intended to invigorate understudies' reasoning and information building.

Content information. Clearly, instructors should know something about the substance they educate. In causing to notice the requirement for more regard for the job of content information in educating, Shulman in 1986 recognized three sorts of content information: topic content information, academic substance information, and curricular information. Topic content information is what a substance expert knows, for instance what a mathematician is familiar with science. Educational substance information is specific information needed for showing the subject, for example, understanding how key thoughts in arithmetic are probably going to be misjudged by students, and different approaches to addressing significant thoughts in the space. Curricular information is information on materials and assets for showing specific substance, including how topic content is organized and sequenced in various materials.

Early examination looked for yet neglected to lay out a reasonable connection between educators' topic information as estimated by how much course-work, grades, and tests-and showing viability; taking greater college science courses didn't be guaranteed to make one a superior instructor of math. In any case, when specialists analyzed what was realized and consequently known by educators, they had the option to lay out an association between the level of disciplinary information and educating viability. As a general rule, instructors with rich topic information will quite often stress calculated, critical thinking, and request parts of their subjects; less educated educators will more often than not underscore realities, rules, and systems. Less educated instructors might adhere near definite plans or the course reading, some of the time missing opportunities to zero in on significant thoughts and associations with different thoughts. At the point when the objective is cultivating understudy understanding and significant learning, as advanced by numerous U.S. instructive change endeavors of the 1980s and 1990s, the requests on an instructor's substance information heighten. Assisting understudies with understanding significant thoughts in a discipline and how these thoughts can be use in differed settings expects that an educator knows more than current realities, ideas, and systems they are instructing. They should likewise know how these thoughts associate with each other and to different spaces.

Frequently, when one considers understanding a discipline-like math, science, or history-one method knowing significant ideas and standards in the field, how they are connected with each other, and how they associate with thoughts in different spaces. Moreover, to be genuinely learned, or "educated," in a specific field includes knowing how specialists in that field think. Knowing science, for instance, involves realizing something about rules for proof and how logical information is laid out. Realizing writing includes understanding what makes a decent evaluate or contention about a scholarly point. To educate particular disciplines well, an educator should know about these parts of disciplinary information and have the option to make them unequivocal in manners that are available to students.

Nature and Form of Teacher Knowledge

A likely risk in depicting different classifications of information for educating is coming to consider educators' information itself coordinated into unique, discrete classifications. Truth be told, what educators know is unpredictably entwined with other information and convictions and with the particular settings where instructors work. Various researchers have presented builds to attempt to catch the complex contextualized nature of instructors' information. A few scientists have contended that educators' characters and valuable encounters assume a significant part in forming the sort of information they foster about educating, referring to this information as "individual functional information." In 1987 Kathy Carter and Walter Doyle contended that a lot of what experienced instructors know is "occasion organized information"- information coordinated around the exercises and occasions they have encountered in homerooms. Others have contended for the significance of articulating the "make information" of instructing the certain speculations, abilities, and approaches to seeing that instructors foster through their work.

In the late 20th and mid twenty-first hundreds of years, such endeavors to understand knowledge for educating have met and been educated by a broader development in brain research and training to see information and discernment as arranged. Simulative scholars place that how and where an individual learns a specific arrangement of information and abilities become a central piece of what is realized. A singular's information is entwined with the physical and social settings where it was gained. These endeavors to describe the manners by which information for instructing is entwined with settings, others, and individual chronicles assist one with valuing the rich and complex nature of what educators need to be aware. Various significant ramifications emerge from this work.

What educators know and how they realize it are attached to specific settings. Creating aptitude in showing involves working and learning with regards to educating. Quite a bit of what educators know is associated with specific devices like course books and educational materials. Quite a bit of what instructors know is routinized and programmed. Similarly, as an individual driving a vehicle with a manual transmission isn't aware of the coordination of developments of feet and hands as they drive-except if an issue emerges a lot of how educators cooperate with understudies is similarly guided by schedule. It is having quite a bit of what they know implanted in these schedules that empowers educators and understudies to oversee in a profoundly perplexing social climate. A drawback of a lot of educators' information being routinized and programmed is that it tends to be challenging to inspect and change when wanted.

Educator Thinking

As mental points of view moved from conduct to mental during the 1970s, various specialists started to zero in on the reasoning cycles involved in educating. A lot of this exploration zeroed in on educators' preparation and navigation. Research on arranging proposes that it happens at various levels (e.g., across a year, across a unit, across a day), that it is for the most part casual (i.e., formal composed plans play to a lesser degree a job than does casual pondering what to do), and that arranging requires an expansive information base (i.e., of the different classes examined previously). Research that zeroed in on the choices made during intelligent showing itself found that educators settled on couple of choices as they instructed and that those choices managed keeping arranged exercises on target. Other examination proposes, nonetheless, that the deep rooted schedules that instructors and understudies have created do a lot to decide the idea of guidance and limit cognizant on-the-spot independent direction.

Figuring out how TO TEACH

The significance of the expression figuring out how to educate appears to be clear and direct, yet as a matter of fact, its definition raises a large group of experimental, reasonable, and regularizing questions. What is it that educators need to be aware, care about, and have the option to do to show actually in various settings? How do instructors fabricate areas of strength for a training and foster an expert personality over the long run? Which job should educator schooling play in figuring out how to educate? How do the states of showing shape the substance of instructor learning? How do perspectives on helping shape speculations of figuring out how to educate?

Figuring out how to instruct is an arising need for policymakers and instructive reformers. For instance, the report of the National Commission on Teaching and America's Future, gave in 1996, put educator learning at the core of its exhaustive outline for change. The report attests that what understudies realize is straightforwardly connected with what instructors educate, and what educators educate relies upon the information, abilities, and responsibilities they bring to their instructing.

Legends About Learning to Teach

The standard way of thinking about figuring out how to educate is established in friendly perspectives toward educating and the experience of being an understudy. A portion of these thoughts contain misleading statements; some have impacted instructive strategy.

Instructors are conceived, not made. Certain individuals trust that the capacity to instruct is a characteristic enrichment like being melodic. A few educators appear to be "naturals" and a few scholars place an intrinsic propensity in people to make sense of things. Indeed, even the organizers behind the normal school accepted that educating was "ladies' actual calling" since it tapped their sense for sustaining the youthful. In any case, the conviction that educators are conceived, not made lays on a thin perspective on the scholarly and individual prerequisites of instructing. It disregards the developing comprehension of instructing as a perplexing, dubious practice, and limits the job of expert schooling in light of the fact that the act of educating can't be educated.

Assuming you know your subject, you can educate it. Whatever else instructors need to be aware, they need to know their subjects. There are educators whose plentiful information and love of their subject make them very compelling despite the fact that they have had no unique groundwork for instructing. Different educators who have broad topic information can't present this information obviously or help other people learn it. Research is starting to explain knowing one's subject for motivations behind showing it, and why traditional measures of subject matter information are hazardous.

By and large, a human sciences instruction was viewed as adequate groundwork for showing optional school. Strategies that require scholarly majors for both rudimentary and optional showing up-and-comers address a contemporary minor departure from this topic. There is mounting proof of educators with a significant in their subject not having the option to make sense of principal ideas in that subject; this present circumstance brings up issues about such strategies.

Researchers have recognized three components of topic information for educating: information on focal realities, ideas, hypotheses and systems; information on logical structures that coordinate and associate thoughts inside a given field; and information on the guidelines of proof and verification in a given field. How is a proof in science not quite the same as a memorable clarification or a scholarly translation? Furthermore, educators should have the option to take a gander at their subjects through the eyes of understudies, guessing what understudies could see as troublesome or befuddling, outlining convincing purposes for concentrating on specific substance, and understanding how thoughts interface across fields and connect with daily existence.

Future educators are probably not going to obtain this sort of information in scholarly courses.

Instructor training gets ready individuals to educate. Though the past fantasies reflect significant wariness about educator training, this fantasy reflects certainty that pre-administration programs get ready individuals to instruct. The normal program comprises of a two-year grouping of instruction courses and field encounters. Normal parts incorporate instructive brain science, general and subject explicit strategies, and understudy educating. What these parts comprise of differs across organizations.

A few examinations show that instructor training is a feeble mediation contrasted and the mingling impacts of educators own rudimentary and optional tutoring, and the impact of hands on experience. Different investigations recommend that serious, reasonable educator training programs really do have an effect. Indeed, even the best program, notwithstanding, can't set someone up to show in a specific setting. The absolute most significant things educators need to know are nearby and must be learned in setting. Pre-administration readiness can establish a groundwork for this complicated, circumstance explicit work, yet the early long stretches of educating are a serious and developmental stage by and by of figuring out how to instruct.

Gradually eases in Learning to Teach

It is difficult to say while figuring out how to educate starts. Since the beginning, individuals are encircled by showing with respect to guardians and educators, and these early encounters with power figures unwittingly shape instructors' educational inclinations. The experience of rudimentary and optional tutoring has an especially impressive effect. From a very long time of instructor watching, planned educators structure pictures of instructing, learning, and topic that impact their future practice except if proficient training mediates.

Liberal examinations influence the manner in which educators contemplate information and move toward the instructing of scholastic substance, albeit not generally in educative headings. At their best, instruction courses and handle encounters develop an expert comprehension of and direction toward educating. Figuring out how to show starts vigorously when beginners step into their own study hall and take up the obligations of full-time educating.

Endeavors to portray the stages educators go through in figuring out how to instruct generally posit an underlying phase of endurance and revelation, a second phase of trial and error and combination, and a third phase of dominance and adjustment. These stages are freely attached to long stretches of involvement, with adjustment happening around the fifth year of educating. Self-information is a significant result of early educating. Beginners make an expert personality through their battles with and investigations of understudies and topic. Over the long haul, educators foster informative schedules and homeroom techniques and gain what's in store from their understudies. Experience by and large yields more noteworthy self-assurance, adaptability, and a feeling of expert independence. Following five to seven years most educators feel they know how to instruct. Whether we refer to these educators as "bosses" or "specialists" relies upon what sort of showing is esteemed and how dominance and ability are characterized.

Models of instructor improvement act as a wakeup call that the method involved with figuring out how to instruct stretches out over various years; in any case, the ongoing design of expert schooling and the states of starting educating don't mirror this. Congruity of learning amazing open doors between pre-administration readiness and new educator acceptance is uncommon. The task of starting educators doesn't mirror their status as students. Most starting instructors have similar obligations as their more experienced partners, and frequently get the most troublesome classes since they need status.

The ascent of formal enlistment programs flags an acknowledgment with respect to an instructors and policymakers that figuring out how to educate happens during the early long stretches of educating. Around thirty states have emotionally supportive networks for starting educators and most metropolitan areas offer some enlistment support, typically as tutor instructors. In any case, not many projects lay on a vigorous comprehension of educator learning or assist fledglings with learning the sort of aggressive educating upheld by reformers. Many projects treat enlistment as momentary help intended to slide the fledgling into full-time instructing.

What could a formative educational program for figuring out how to instruct involve? Which undertakings have a place with introductory planning and which to the enlistment stage? In spite of holes in information and an absence of agreement about the most effective ways to plan educators and backing their learning after some time, conceptualizing a continuum of learning potential open doors for teachers is conceivable.

Instructor Preparation and Learning to Teach

Assuming educators are to gain proficiency with a rendition of instructing that they have not experienced as students, they need to foster new edges of reference for deciphering what goes on in homerooms and coming to conclusions about what and how to educate. Situated between educators' previous experience as understudies and their future experience as educators, college based instructor training is very much arranged to empower this change in thinking. Except if pre-administration instructors reproduce their initial convictions about educating, learning, understudies, and topic, proceeding with experience will set these convictions, making them even less helpless to change.

A second undertaking of educator planning especially fit to college based study is assisting future instructors with creating reasonable and educational information on their educating subjects. Current instructive changes have provoked reestablished interest in educators' topic information since they require a sort of instructing that connects with understudies in obtaining information, yet additionally in building and conveying about information. This undertaking relies upon commitments from expressions and sciences, and schooling.

To construct spans between topic and understudies, educators should comprehend what kids resemble at various ages, how they figure out their reality, how their perspectives and acting are molded by their language and culture, how they gain information and abilities, and foster certainty as students. This foundation information turns out to be progressively basic as educators work with kids whose racial, social, and financial foundations contrast from their own.

To gain from educating, educator competitors should foster the fundamental devices and demeanors. This incorporates abilities of perception, understanding and investigation, the propensity for supporting cases about understudy learning with proof, the eagerness to think about elective clarifications. In the event that educator competitors work on these abilities with others, they might start to consider partners to be assets in figuring out how to instruct.

In spite of the fact that educators need to know numerous things, compelling training relies upon the capacity to utilize information properly specifically circumstances. Pre-administration educators can start fostering a collection of ways to deal with educational program, guidance, and evaluation during pre-administration readiness. Figuring out how to adjust and involve this information practically speaking is a proper assignment for educator acceptance.

Instructor Induction and Learning to Teach

Enlistment occurs regardless of a proper program; nonetheless, the presence of a solid program can limit the endurance mindset that grasps such countless starting educators and situate their learning in useful headings. Starting educators need to become familiar with the objectives and guidelines for understudies at their grade level, and how these assumptions fit into a bigger structure of educational program and evaluation. They should get to know their understudies and local area, and sort out some way to involve this information in fostering a responsive educational plan.

On the off chance that instructor planning has been fruitful, starting educators will have a dream of good instructing and a starting collection reliable with that vision. A significant undertaking for starting instructors is obtaining the neighborhood understandings and fostering the adaptability of reaction to institute this collection. The difficulties of educating alone interestingly can deter new educators from attempting aggressive teaching methods. Acceptance backing can hold them back from leaving such methodologies for what they see as more secure, less perplexing exercises. It can likewise assist tenderfoots with zeroing in on the reasons and in addition to the administration of learning exercises and their importance for understudies.

To show in manners that answer understudies and push learning ahead, educators should have the option to evoke and decipher understudies' thoughts and produce fitting showing moves as the example unfurls. Paying attention to what understudies say and building reactions on a second to-second premise; and taking care of the necessities of the gathering while at the same time taking care of people requires impressive expertise and practice: It addresses a requesting learning task for starting instructors. Starting educators should make and keep a homeroom learning local area that is protected, conscious, and useful of understudy learning. Issues of force and control lie at the core of this undertaking that is restricted with learners' advancing proficient character. Frequently starting instructors battle to accommodate contending pictures of their job as they develop a reasonable expert position.

Assuming instructors are asked the way in which they figured out how to educate, they will say they figured out how to instruct by educating. In spite of the fact that experience assumes a significant part in figuring out how to educate, there is a major distinction between "having" experience and learning desirable examples from that experience. To gain from the experience of educating, instructors should have the option to involve their training as a site for request. This implies transforming disarrays into questions, exploring different avenues regarding new methodologies and concentrating on the impacts, and outlining new inquiries to broaden their comprehension.

The continuous review and improvement of educating is hard to achieve alone. Educators need potential chances to consult with others about instructing, to break down examples of understudy work, to look at curricular materials, to examine issues and think about various clarifications and activities. Numerous reformers accept that this sort of scholarly work can best be achieved by gatherings of educators cooperating over the long haul.

Techniques FOR STUDYING

Showing has been the subject of efficient request for a considerable length of time. The principal American Educational Research Association Handbook of Research on Teaching, altered by Nathaniel L. Gage, showed up in 1963 and later releases have showed up at roughly ten-year stretches. Since the 1960s there have likewise been various huge surveys of this examination, like Arnold Morrison and Donald McIntyre's 1969 and 1973 releases of Teachers and Teaching and Penelope L. Peterson and Herbert J. Walberg's Research on Teaching (1979). Such surveys have featured both the intricacy of educating and the way that it is manageable to study from various viewpoints, utilizing different techniques.

Investigation into showing has been sought after for basically three unique purposes. To begin with, specialists and experts intend to see better the cycles in question, to foster the information base of instructing, and to add to hypothetical structures, which help to conceptualize educating. Second, inquiry into educating has likewise been sought after for the motivations behind further developing practice. This is especially the situation, for example, in real life research concentrates on that for the most part follow a cycle, starting with the ID of a functional issue or area of concern, trailed by the get-together of proof utilizing different exploration techniques, choices about how to change practice, and afterward the social event of additional proof to screen the impacts of the change. Such cycles are regularly rehashed and give a method for continually observing and further developing practice as well as fostering an upgraded self-basic mindfulness. Third, request is characteristic for proficient arrangement, and exploration strategies might be utilized by understudy educators, for instance, in assisting with getting a handle on their perceptions of educating and in fostering their own training. Homeroom association plans, for instance, have oftentimes been utilized to help understudy educators to structure their perceptions and to take note of the manners by which instructors get clarification on some pressing issues, or move starting with one errand then onto the next inside the homeroom, or manage understudy conduct issues. Any one examination project, notwithstanding, might be being sought after for any of these reasons and could draw upon a wide range of exploration strategies to accomplish its points.

Research Methods

Different techniques have been utilized to assemble data about educating. The most widely recognized fall into the accompanying classes: methodical perception, contextual analysis and ethnography, study procedures, recreations, critiques, idea planning, and accounts. Each yields its own particular sort of information about educating, and might be pretty much suitable for various purposes as examined underneath.

Orderly perception. Ned Flanders in 1970 was quick to promote the utilization of perception plans for the investigation of educating. His Flanders Interaction Analysis Categories (FIAC) distinguished ten classifications of conduct that portrayed educator understudy association inside the study hall. Eyewitnesses, when prepared in recognizing and sorting these ways of behaving, could then code their perceptions, which would later be read up for communication designs. Flanders' work has since been explained with various timetables intended for explicit purposes. Perception plans basically give an agenda of ways of behaving that the specialist is keen on, and empower an example of educators' connections to be portrayed in quantitative terms.

Once in a while the timetable is more situated towards concentrating on a grouping of showing conduct as opposed to the amount of various kinds of conduct and might be utilized to distinguish the manners by which ways of behaving change after some time or because of an exploratory mediation.

The significant benefit of efficient perception is that it gives a moderately genuine record of homeroom conduct. For example, it could portray the extent of inquiries that an educator pose to that are unassuming, or the proportion of instructor orders that have a disciplinary concentration, or the overall number of times that instructors or understudies start connection. The strategy, in any case, is seldom ready to offer a lot of data about the setting of specific communications, and can't enlighten the translations that educators and understudies place upon their own and others' way of behaving. An inquiry coordinated toward an understudy, for example, might involve basic review for one, a mentally difficult errand for another, a to a great extent friendly trade in one setting or a suggested censure in an alternate setting, and the spectator might not be able to recognize adequate signals to see the value in completely its importance. Efficient perception might be helpful, consequently, in taking into account the general effect of new educational program materials on educational way of behaving, for instance, however may have restricted esteem on its own in recognizing the full intricacies of educators' work, why instructors act as they do, and the thinking that directs their activities.

Contextual investigation and ethnography. Some have contended that contextual analysis and ethnography allude more to ways to deal with research than strategies in themselves. Habitually they draw upon meetings and semi-organized perceptions, though occasionally on other proof too, to come to a comprehension of a specific educator's training. One of their distinctive highlights is that they include in-depth study. Over an extensive timeframe, the specialist can see the value in the setting in which an educator works, and through collaboration with the instructor about their training can form bits of knowledge into how they view their work. These experiences can then be tried against future perceptions or different information. Gaea Leichardt

(1988), for instance, noticed a few science examples showed by one instructor and talked with her finally both about her educating and about her previous encounters of math. Thus, she had the option to sort out a comprehension of the manners by which the educator's own learning of science as an understudy and her encounters of expert preparation had come to impact her way to deal with showing the subject. Contextual analyses have every now and again featured the manners by which educators adapt to the complex contending requests that they face in their work or the manners by which starting educators experience and defeat the underlying challenges of figuring out how to educate.

Contextual investigations and ethnographies regularly include the examination of exceptionally a lot of subjective information, and an essayist definitely stand out to the likelihood that specialists can separate from these their own specific translations. The capability of ethnographic examination to yield speculations about educating has likewise been discussed, for certain analysts contending that the value of the methodology lies in the bits of knowledge about specific parts of instructing that such investigations can give.

Study strategies. Studies on educators and instructing have depended on the utilization of polls, organized interviews, agendas, tests, or disposition scales. Reviews have been utilized to depict the qualities of educators as an expert gathering, like their perspectives towards kids, their viewpoints about a specific development, or their own yearnings and sensations of occupation fulfillment. They have additionally been utilized to gather educators' own depictions of their practices or the expert worries they have at various phases of their professions.

Studies permit information to be gathered about enormous quantities of educators, and on the off chance that proper testing methods are utilized and an adequately exceptional yield rate is obtained, it is feasible to make speculations about educators overall or about specific gatherings of instructors, like grade teachers, or educators in a specific branch of knowledge or geological locale. Reviews, in any case, can gather data that educators can without much of a stretch report, and different techniques are required in the event that the scientist wishes to enter all the more profoundly into the mind boggling communications of educators' reasoning and conduct and the settings where they work.

Reenactments. An assortment of reenactment methods has been fostered that include giving educators an errand or circumstance like one that would be experienced in their typical work and seeing how efficient varieties in the idea of various undertakings or circumstances influences the manners in which instructors mean to manage them. Such strategies have been utilized to research how educators plan examples, what they are meant for in their dynamic by outside imperatives, or what they are meant for in their cooperation's with understudies by various understudy credits. Mary M. Rohrkemper and Jeer E. Trophy (1983), for instance, furnished educators with depictions or vignettes of kids in a variety of homeroom circumstances, each introducing a specific test to the instructor. By looking at the connection between the educators' decisions or choices and the variables fluctuating inside the vignettes, it was feasible to recognize those elements of kids that are powerful in educators' contemplating issue circumstances. Reenactments can be utilized to evoke the information that educators have and use in their ordinary practice and that may be challenging to access through different strategies.

Analyses. Understanding the cycles of educating includes understanding the significance educator's characteristic to their activities and the reasoning's they have for acting as they do. Endeavors to get to the continuous reasoning and decision-production of educators have required the utilization of strategies especially designed for evoking instructors' information and manners of thinking. This has included verbally process conventions where educators, while participated in a preparation or evaluation task, for instance, have endeavored to express their considerations simultaneously. The reasoning and decision-production of educators during dynamic instructing have been evoked involving invigorated review methods in which an example is recorded and later played back to the educators who endeavor to review their reasoning at that point. A few specialists have likewise utilized the notes taken from perception of examples to structure interviews with educators a short time later to build a discourse on the thing the instructor was doing and the explanations behind their activities.

Research in this space has raised a few issues about the situation with educators' verbal reports on their training: Do they truly mirror educators' genuine reasoning at that point, or would they say they are after-the-occasion supports? What's more, might the idea that accompanies viable activity at any point be satisfactorily addressed as far as words alone, or is "genuine" suspected the same thing restricted with pictures, illustrations, and sentiments? There are a few reasonable issues concerning this sort of exploration strategy, and obviously care should be taken to think about possible wellsprings of twisting in self-report information. By the by, steps can be taken to limit such impacts, and these techniques have been utilized successfully to investigate a portion of the mental parts of educators' work.

Idea planning. A few procedures, inexactly named as idea planning, have been utilized to address' comprehension educators might interpret different parts of their work. They by and large follow a three-stage process, starting with conceptualizing on a specific subject to distinguish ideas, trailed by a course of showing how these ideas are interrelated, lastly naming the connections between the ideas. The finished result is a visual portrayal of educators' comprehension as it connects with a specific subject. Greta Morine-Dershimer (1991), for instance, utilized the procedure to recognize the manners by which different understudy educators ponder homeroom the board: some understudy instructors, for instance, would link classroom the executives to ideas of individual connections, study hall environment, and an ethos of common regard, though others would interface it to ideas of rules, endorses, rewards, and acclaim. Such strategies can assist with enlightening the various understandings that understudy educators hold of key ideas or might be utilized to distinguish the progressions that happen in instructors' understandings over the long haul or because of in-service preparing or educational plan advancement.

Accounts. Story concentrates on expect to give a record of showing in a way that would sound natural to educators. They support an experiential way to deal with depicting educators' work, taking specific note of the instructors' "voice" and putting educators' insight inside the setting of other life altering situations. Account scientists have much of the time contended against additional unthinking ways to deal with depicting educating and have contended for a narrating approach in which the specialist goes about as a facilitator assisting educators with relating their involvement in due acknowledgment of the individual and context oriented factors inside which it is outlined. D. Jean Clendenin (1986), for instance, creates story of three essential educators. Every story features a vital picture or directing similitude that is persuasive in molding the educator's opinion on educating and learning. One educator, for example, held animate of "language as the key" and language was seen as the premise of all homeroom action. One more held the picture of "study hall as home" and this picture showed itself in her associations with kids and in her association of the homeroom. In 1994 J. Gary Knowles, Arora L. Cole, and Colleen S. Press wood outlined the challenges of understudy instructors on field insight through the development of stories, drawing to a great extent on the understudies own personal histories, journals, and conversations. This way to deal with research has filled quickly as of late and has animated a few discussions about the status and veracity of stories.

End

Research on educating has involved a great many various techniques. Each enjoys its own benefits as well as its disadvantages. Each can possibly enlighten specific parts of the instructing system. Various strategies are proper for various inquiries. Besides, certain directions towards research, for example, mental or experiential-incline analysts toward specific sorts of request and therefore specific techniques. Educating, be that as it may, is a mind boggling process and the rich and various methods of request presently accessible empower specialists to seek after those intricacies and to completely add to their seeing more.

A regular perspective on instructing holds that it requires something like Mark Hopkins, a kid, and a log. Presence of mind lets us know we might shed the log however that two individuals, not be guaranteed to man and kid, are fundamental. Further, there should be a comprehension between the two that one finds out about something than the other and ought to confer it. As per this view, the demonstration of educating is a basic cycle: it is to give or bestow information.

The regular view furnishes us with a conceivable model. It recommends well known thoughts of what might turn out badly: unfortunate educating happens when educators have too little information or too little expertise to bestow the information they have. However, the model isn't fulfilling. In alluding just to the educator, it dismisses the collaboration of instructor and student, and it neglects to make sense of the general, if discontinuous, obstruction of understudies, the antagonism, once in a while exchanging with reverence and love, so frequently coordinated at educators.

For there is struggle in educating; it is a strain filled, chancy cycle. Protection from educating happens among students who are capable and restless to learn; it happens when instructors instruct well. It isn't bound to schools however regularly happens in the casual showing circumstances of day to day existence, as everybody realizes who has attempted to help a companion to drive a vehicle.

We can move toward comprehension of one wellspring of the contention among instructor and student in the event that we consider helping an endeavor to change the understudy by acquainting him with groundbreaking thoughts. In this model, educating is an attack on oneself, and protection from it tends to be cleared up as reluctance for upset one's inward business as usual. Conceivable as it might appear, the model is by and by restricted in application. It enlightens the intriguing case: the understudy adequately mindful of the force of thoughts to dread and battle them, the student with an energetic and influential instructor of a subject loaded with thoughts of the sort that open new universes of comprehension of self. It doesn't make sense of the substantially more typical instance of the careless, unconcerned student who has a dull instructor of a dry subject. Yet, it is plausible that there is so a lot, while perhaps not more, struggle among educator and student in the last option case than in the previous. We want a model of instructing that fits a wide range of understudies, educators, and subjects.

A contention model of instructing. In each showing circumstance, the educator is, at least for a brief time, the unrivaled and his student the subordinate, a relationship we might communicate in prepositional structure as follows: A (the predominant) starts connection for B (the subordinate), and B answers as per A's desires; all the more just, a provides orders that B complies (Humans 1950, p. 244). From the prevalent point of view, this assertion portrays what is happening in which his capacity to control B's reaction is unchallenged — an ideal not accomplished all the time. At the point when control is unsure, the best assumes the power of commitment: if A doesn't control B's reaction, he ought to; as predominant, it is his obligation.

We can apply this contingent type of Humans' recommendation to instructing. As educator, a starts connection for B by granting information or guiding him to it. Simultaneously, an acknowledges the commitment to make sure that B answers as he (A) wishes. In satisfying his obligation, an assesses the rightness of B's reaction and controls B's way of behaving during the communication adequately to make right reaction conceivable. Basically, A's job is that of order and B's of accommodation.

While not unavoidable, struggle among educator and understudy is unsurprising in this model (Waller [1932] 1961, p. 195). The nonappearance, instead of the presence, of opposition requires clarification when one individual looks for such a lot of command over another. Educating, in this model, is making the understudy learn; and an educator's undertaking is one of so dealing with the contention his endeavors might incite that accommodation is impermanent and the student's soul whole.

Decrease of contention. Our challenges with showing in regular day to day existence recommend that subjection is for sure key to educating. We feel most calm when A's status outside the showing dyad is better than B's. While possibly not in every case happily, youngsters acknowledge educating from their elderly folks, and novices take it from old hands. Subjection turns into an issue, notwithstanding, when an is equivalent or sub-par in status to B. In these conditions, we utilize various gadgets to alleviate struggle. Between companions, what is basically a nonreciprocal relationship can be expressed, "I'll train you to swim, in the event that you instruct me to. . .." Each gets a sense of ownership with the other in this connection, yet not at the same time. We rely upon the guaranteed inversion of job to improve subjection.

In additional organized connections, correspondence might be unimaginable. Circumstances emerge in which one of two people equivalent in rank knows something the other should be aware to carry on his work. At the point when this occurs, the last option might be initiated to request help, with the goal that the educator appears to be less similar to an instructor since he doesn't start the collaboration. "Educating" isn't utilized. All things considered, one partner "assists" another or "helps out." The aide might make a special effort to clarify that he sees himself as better in information than his partner exclusively with regards to this issue in question.

Educating is improper when B has extremely high status. Chiefs of boats are not workable during order, or organization presidents on issues of business. As a matter of fact, it is society intelligence not to attempt to show anybody his business, whatever his position.

At the point when guidance is required, high-positioning individuals utilize an expert on unambiguous issues for which he is approached to outfit answers for be evaluated solely after he has gone. Denied of command over his understudy's learning and of chance to assess it, the expert is less threatening to the one who employs him, however he leaves the scene with an awkward feeling of unfulfilled obligation.

Not utilizing "educating" while educating is being finished, prompting the student to request it, correspondence of job, and severe restriction of the subject matter are gadgets regularly used to keep away from the contention intrinsic in instructing. However, anxiety, in the event that not antagonism, remains. Companion, expert, aide actually feel liable for their understudy's reaction and may attempt to control it. Students should stow away from themselves the information that even in such a shortened relationship they might have uncovered themselves unequipped for right reaction. One can send away the instructor however not before he has taken one's action.

School and study hall

The gadgets that alleviate struggle among educator and student in regular daily existence are only occasionally utilized (in spite of the fact that they might be play-acted) in the schoolroom. The educator's status as a grown-up makes correspondence of job unbelievable, since he can't be set in that frame of mind of kid understudy. In supposed vote based showing techniques, connection might appear to start with the understudy, yet all aside from the most youthful sense the educator's directing hand and as often as possible dislike the misrepresentation (Seeley et al. 1956, p. 271).

An understudy might step up to the plate by requesting assist with an issue, so the educator turns into a mentor expert who goes about as though both he and the student needed to fulfill outside inspectors. Be that as it may, this type of collaboration is essentially rare; regardless of what endeavors school and educators make to show people, a significant part of the day goes on in the lockstep the school's economy of existence requires. The educator converses with every one of his understudies as a unit; he relegates examples and gives assessments to the gathering. On the off chance that there are outside inspectors, he does his own testing and evaluating first. It is just toward the finish of a tutoring succession, when understudies continue on toward another framework, that educator and class join endeavors to pass assessments.

Authority of the instructor. In regular showing circumstances, we limit possible struggle by restricting the educator's power or imagining it doesn't exist. Schools do the inverse. They support and real his clout in various ways. The instructor enjoys the benefit of his own ground — the independent unit of the homeroom and the encasing walls of the school building, what cut the understudy off from the remainder of his reality. The educator has reliable partners another instructor, the school organization, and the state. His strategies for control and assessment (discipline and evaluating) get institutional help in the record keeping of the organization. While there might be misconceptions among these partners of the instructor and weakness to outside pressures, they enjoy the benefit of being grown-ups managing youngsters. They keep a proceeding with control in which the understudy is consistently dependent upon the power of an educator, in a school the law expects him to join in.

The school additionally supports the educator's power by legitimating his cases to information. It guarantees the local area that its educators have scholastic degrees and experience. Moreover, the teacher manages information frameworks that have a goal character naturally separate from the individual of both the instructor and the understudy (Simmel 1950, p. 132). Educator and understudy don't just concur, as in casual instructing, that the educator has unrivaled information; it involves public agreement that he does.

With such countless partners thus much help of his power, the educator's position seems unassailable. In the event that there is to be a few type of contention among him and his understudies, he should clearly win. Understudies are not vulnerable, nonetheless. Their folks might intervene, and the law as a rule precludes whipping. In the study hall they enjoy the extraordinary benefit of being numerous to the educator's one. Like any gathering, students can better their condition by acting together to tackle normal issues, and a unified class furnishes an instructor with a considerable rival.

In rigorously run schools, be that as it may, where grades are of essential significance, the educator frequently maintains a strategic distance from struggle among himself and his understudies by empowering struggle among the actual students. He keeps students from participating in aggregate activity against him by prompting them to contend with one another in classwork. He has every understudy recount to him as opposed to the class and maintains the fiction that learning happens honestly just inside the dyad of educator and student. At the point when an educator structures cooperation in the homeroom along these lines, understudies are exceptionally mindful that they offer a similar item to an educator whose central job is that of evaluator of items. In any case, as Marshall ([1963] 1965, pp. 181-183) notes, closeness need not partition; contenders frequently become accomplices. At the point when they do, another type of contention creates, in which students join to deal with the educator about the conditions of their participation with him. In present day libertarian social orders, where educators frequently feel awkward in a tyrant job and despise contest for grades, haggling is presumably the most continuous type of contention among instructor and understudies.

Bartering among educator and understudies. The way that the school's economy requires the educator to regard his class as a unit in many, while possibly not all, regards without a doubt works with the improvement of agreement and aggregate activity with respect to understudies or, as it has somewhere else been designated, "understudy culture" (Becker et al. 1961, pp. 435-437). The term assigns an inconspicuous utilization of the financial specialist's gadget of restricting the region of the educator's mastery. This understudy activity is a drive for a smidgen of independence communicated in dealing with the educator about issues he doesn't ordinarily characterize as instructing however for which he by the by feels mindful: control of the student's way of behaving during learning.

By listening cautiously to what an educator says he needs in class and comparing among themselves what grades or remarks he gives for what sorts of work, and by "giving things a shot" (mass shoestring tying, for example) in the beginning of a school term, a class might arrive at an agreement about its instructor's norms, both scholar and disciplinary. It then changes what the educator says and does into rules for him to keep. He should not change these standards the class makes for him, and he should apply them to all students.

It doesn't make any difference much the way that high an instructor sets norms of calm, tidiness of work, or instantaneousness, in spite of the fact that there will be fights assuming that his guidelines are off the mark with those of different educators. What is important is consistency of use. According to his understudies, this is the instructor's essential for the deal. On the off chance that it isn't kept, he can anticipate inconvenience. Educators who neglect to figure out the essential reason — "We will act appropriately, assuming you act appropriately" — end up ceaselessly taken part in restraining students as opposed to granting information.

A portion of the guidelines of the deal understudies make with an educator are in that hazy situation constantly dependent upon exchange — levels of tidiness or quietness, for instance. Different guidelines are obvious: an educator may not give a test on things not in the text or on issues not shrouded in class. Rules change from one study hall to another and starting with one school then onto the next, obviously, and with the age and refinement of students. However, wherever the to a great extent implicit deal his students make with him obliges the educator's way of behaving regardless of whether he knows it.

Students have compelling approvals which they use to compensate and rebuff instructors who neglect to satisfy the deal, sanctions not many educators can endure. On one day, when a guest comes, they please the educator with model way of behaving; on the following, they create a ruckus in the homeroom that is clearly sufficient to reverberate in the ears of the head, the guardians, and the whole local area. Subject to his understudies' kindness and collaboration, the instructor before long consents to the bartering practices of the class, frequently entering the game for his own sake. According to he, as a result, "In the event that you will hush up, you might possess more energy for the test"; by this activity he perceives and consequently reinforces the collectivity as well as endures illegal scholastic practice to get discipline.

The deal likewise characterizes the instructor's locale. Understudies concur that in his study hall the educator may really control the scholar (illustrations and tests), endeavor to control the semi intellectual (note passing and pencil honing), and fairly allude the nonacademic (dress and ethics) to the seriously enveloping power of the head. In students' eyes, notwithstanding, consistently the scholarly legitimizes an educator's control. Passages, washrooms, and yards are spatially eliminated from books and study; the educator controls them as he can.

The educator isn't probably going to see the rationale of these differentiations. That's what he knows whether he is to control one understudy's scholarly reaction in the homeroom, control of the entire class is an essential, and that control of the class relies on the discipline of contiguous rooms and corridors. The school organization, seeking after its regulatory course, additionally finds conduct inconsequential to the scholastic threatening to the smooth working of the school and to its standing. As consequence, the dress, habits, and ethics (at times the groups of understudies on account of less advantaged gatherings) become subject matters and endeavored control. In certain schools, educators and organization legitimize the expansion by declaring liability, hard to understand, over the "entire kid." It frequently is in such evidently irrelevant issues as legitimate dress that dealing among educator and understudies separates, opening the way to different types of a third type of contention — revolt.

Whatever its structure — rivalry among students that the educator should cautiously propagate, bartering in which he should share, or revolts he should put down — struggle is challenging for the educator who sticks to the regular thought that his only capability is one of giving information. On the off chance that he considers himself an unrivaled controlling the way of behaving of numerous uncontrollable subordinates, he may ultimately come to partake in the fight.

Preparing establishments for educators

Educators' schools and college schools of instruction supply the school system with workers and offer with it the long-range objective of teaching the youthful. Considering this cozy relationship, we could anticipate that preparing establishments should plan educators for struggle with understudies, however they don't. All things considered, they follow the regular model with which we started: to instruct is to confer or offer information. Would-be instructors learn topic and methods of educating. They step through courses in examination development and translation, however testing isn't perceived as a gadget for controlling understudies, and discipline (control of a collectivity) is only sometimes thought to be a legitimate subject of guidance. Spur of the moment, such disjunction between the ordinary work of an occupation and the preparation one gets for it appears to be uncommon. However, any place preparing is isolated from training (or, in other words, any place there are schools), we track down a comparable circumstance. Most schools instruct a lot of that is rarely utilized and neglect to show what is.

We might make sense of the disjunction by alluding to the situational points of view (sets of convictions and activities) of the different gatherings in the preparation organization that together make up its way of life. Individuals in both the schools and the preparation establishments for educator's foster approaches to acting, objectives, and interests in response to the specific issues presented by their circumstance (Becker et al. 1961, pp. 34-37). Schools and educators' universities are both piece of the bigger order of instructive organizations committed to a shared objective, however their quick circumstances vary.

While school individuals should manage nearby legislative issues, neighborhoods (great and awful), guardians, and other vested parties, educators' universities exist in a scholastic setting different in situational goals and imperatives. Theirs is the universe of schools and colleges so able to concede esteem, with every one of its honors, generally to the academic disciplines. Since the regular model of educating accentuates information, it fits the scholastic world better than the contention model with its emphasis on interactive abilities. Resources of training might be "school-reared" — numerous establishments expect teachers to have shown in the state funded schools (Hughes 1963a, p. 152) — yet the pattern in such resources throughout the years is toward a looser bind with the schools. Put aside on his grounds with his more significant salary and status, the educator of instructors moves away from instructors of kids. His foundation may officially mirror the association of the educational system by its division into special, elementary, and secondary school projects, and state authorizing guidelines might set the grouping of understudies' courses; yet these articulating gadgets tend more to limit development by both preparation school and understudy than to carry future instructors nearer to the contention vital to instructing.

Enrolling. The disjunction of preparing and work, which forestalls the transmission of helpfully precise information on what's in store in a genuine showing circumstance, without a doubt helps the educational system to enroll youthful educators. It is feasible to fill showing position considerably under states of deficiency, yet the schools maintain that should accomplish more than fill them. Like other help foundations and organizations, they need volunteers of high capacity focused on a lifetime vocation. In a word, they need experts.

Tragically, understudies of the greatest capacity only from time to time enter preparing foundations for educators (Vereen 1961), and not all graduates instruct (Osborn and Maul 1961). There are amazing purposes behind this. Of the glad old purposes for living, instructing requires the most un-formal schooling and thusly minimal speculation of time, money, and energy. The institute of training gives a somewhat un-explicit school program that can cause no damage. To enter preparing is in no sense a guarantee to a profession. For would-be competitors, performers, and specialists dubious of progress as entertainers and for ladies whose best option of profession is marriage, a degree in schooling is a type of word related protection.

In spite of the fact that educating is exceptionally apparent to kids from the get-go in their lives, the openness isn't probably going to draw in them to the occupation. The educator is an over the top day to day bad guy to create, for instance, the moly of the doctor who comes to help the family in difficult situation. For offspring of manual laborers, educating may convey renown; yet for those of higher social starting points, appearing to be a hard life for the reward is more probable. As a lady's occupation, it likewise bears the disgrace (for the two genders) of lady's low status in correlation with men; yet it isn't sufficiently female, besides at the nursery level, to firmly draw in ladies.

Individuals who really do enter instructing find that in correlation with different occupations startlingly ailing in the helper rewards work with responsibility (Becker 1960). Industry and business offer advancement to additional capable situations, while school showing offers just salary raises and inconsequential status honors. Educators leave the study hall, obviously, to become trained professionals or executives; yet as lengthy they keep on instructing, there is little an open door for the more-than-nearby impact conceivable in different callings through distribution, addressing, and discussion.

Despite the fact that educators manage individuals instead of with things (an old status differentiation), individuals they manage are minors. They miss the prizes, mental and political, of serving individuals of high status and power. Their day to day work is frequently customized by state divisions of education; no teachers oversee and guide them in manners which make the independence valued by conventional experts and business people unimaginable. Under such circumstances, we ought not be astonished that the selecting of committed experts is troublesome.

Vocation and calling

When begun a showing vocation, the disjunction between their planning and reality in the schools frequently hits educators hard. Looked as they are every day with threatening kids on and on expecting more prominent independence, we might ask why any of them proceed. Without a trace of exploration, we can guess, yet it is likely that many individuals wind up focused on instructing on the grounds that a best option profession bombs them. The ideal marriage or acknowledgment in some universe of sports, writing, or craftsmanship won't ever emerge. Educators may likewise commit themselves accidentally on the grounds that the occupation licenses different inclusions. For a wedded man, low compensation might require working two jobs, and this subsequent work, fitted to a showing plan, may turn out to be remunerating to such an extent that he keeps on educating. Hitched ladies who find that showing fits well with family and youngster raising obligations may likewise go on in educating.

There is, likewise, the security of residency and, every now and again, bliss in latency. School undertakings endlessly rehash; many years the round is something similar. One may become so set apart by drenching in the realm of a ghetto school that one feels unfitted for some other (Becker 1952, p. 474). Obligation to people is decreased by the steady turnover of students who sit in one's group for a year and are gone. In time, expecting control of a class might become pleasant. A portion of the very things about instructing that deter beginners might keep veterans at it (Geer 1966).

Educators as experts. All the more decidedly, individuals might concede to educating on the grounds that it is, in many regards, a calling. Educators can't guarantee the different character given by control of a recondite assortment of information (Hughes 1963b, p. 657), yet they in all actuality do have the obscure abilities of the homeroom. They don't have proficient social orders sufficiently able to shield them from the attacks of the local area, guardians, and specialists on training outside the educational system, yet it is for the most part in light of a legitimate concern for the head to safeguard them (Becker 1953, pp. 133-139). They are regulated, however there is as yet something left of the desolate distinction of the study hall. Deceivability of execution is low; and not many individuals accept we have advanced at this point how to gauge showing capacity (Brim1958).

Locally, instructing appears to hold a portion of the more horrendous parts of a calling. There are leftovers of the assumption that educators ought to be models of appropriateness for the youthful; even grown-ups are once in a while humiliated in their demanding presence. The public items to requests for more significant compensation since educators live on citizens' cash. They should serve the local area happily.

Instructors themselves show uncertainty about their status by having associations as well as expert social orders. The last option has little control (despite the fact that they progressively endeavor it) over morals, enlisting, preparing, or regulation influencing educators. They have not yet concluded whether school chairmen and experts ought to be remembered for their relationship as "educators" or kept out as managers and adversaries. Associations assist educators with battling for more significant salary and against the infringements of obligations in schoolyards, lounges, and latrines. Yet, they are more well-suited to bring down that esteem so vital to a minor calling than to increase it.

Educators feel they have an unfortunate public picture and lacking public appreciation, yet for some instructing is a move forward in friendly class and in this way in regard. Huge city frameworks assist educators with getting the extra training expected for specialization and salary increases. Chance to move to the requests ante working circumstances in working class schools accompanies position (Becker 1953). For men, school teaching might be a Band-Aid, if at this point not a venturing stone end route to additional renowned vocations. For ladies, it very well may be a fantastic and, surprisingly, innovative occupation that interferes short of what others upon a spouse and youngsters.

Educators are not experts in the standard sense. They don't have clients who pick them, end the relationship, or bring to it the quick need of help that tempers the client's subjection to the doctor or legal counselor. From a more extensive perspective, they are experts with the general public for client. We can't manage without their transmission, but blemished, of its legacy. It is even likely that society would be very unique had kids no an open door to take part in struggle with their boss, the educator, and consequently no chance to learn early something of the strength that aggregate activity brings to subordinates.

Right now, more is realized about how individuals learn than any other time in mankind's set of experiences, and forward leaps in research are happening with expanding recurrence. The sociologies have contributed tremendously to this assortment of hypothetical information, yet the dissemination of instructive advancements stays dangerous. New hypotheses and practices as a rule don't totally uproot existing teaching methods yet are essentially added to instructors' educational collection. In addition, the interpretation of hypothesis into study hall practice relies on how well individual educators comprehend the speculations they were shown and the way that they set them up as a regular occurrence.

During the 20th century clinicians and instructive scholars fostered a wide assortment of models to make sense of how people learn, and obviously continuous fundamental exploration an affects instructive practice at all levels of the schooling system. Late examination in neuroscience has likewise added a natural aspect to how we might interpret the educational experience, albeit the instructive ramifications of this exploration are as yet not satisfactory.

A few significant topics have risen up out of this group of examination. For instance, there is significant arrangement that for profound figuring out how to happen, students should build new information themselves, through experience, reflection, and coordination. Students likewise should expand on what they definitely know and accept, so they should accommodate existing information with new information and right mixed up convictions. Metacognitive abilities, for example, decisive reasoning and critical thinking, are essential objectives of learning, yet dominance of genuine information is likewise vital for decisive reasoning. Real information is best scholarly inside reasonable systems that coordinate it in significant ways, and since subject disciplines utilize various structures, understudies need to gain proficiency with different methodologies for sorting out their insight.

These hypotheses propose that understudies should take part in learning undertakings that require request, trial and error, and dynamic commitment to genuine critical thinking. Bunch based exercises and undertakings are regularly involved showing techniques in this worldview, since participation and joint effort appear to work with the ideal results. The educator's substance skill is as yet significant; however, it is utilized in original ways. Addressing and discourse generally supplant addressing, and the instructor turns into an educational mentor who plans learning exercises, works with conversation, and guides understudies through the most common way of learning.

With different transformations, these standards can be applied at all degrees of guidance, from youth to grown-up schooling. For instance, in a grade school, understudies use models of the sun, the earth, and the moon, and a splendid light to lead a trial to make sense of the periods of the moon. Toward the finish of the activity, they review their determinations and step through an examination on the fundamental cosmic ideas. In a school science course, understudy bunches are given a contextual investigation on stream contamination. They work cooperatively to pool their natural information, suggest researchable conversation starters, foster a learning plan that incorporates readings for the gathering, lead an examination of the inquiries, lastly produce experimentally solid arrangements. The result of their work is assessed on the exactness of their insight, the painstakingness of their examination, and the nature of their logical thinking.

Albeit experimental examination obviously upholds the viability of these academic methodologies, just the most moderate instructive organizations advance and backing them as the essential method of guidance. Normally, chose exercises and tasks happen just inconsistently inside the setting of traditional didactic guidance. The reasons these hypotheses have not been more unavoidable in training are connected with a portion of the essential issues of making an interpretation of hypothesis into training.

Past the troubles of dominating new educational strategies and procedures, educators frequently find it hard to forsake the job of master did act and the informative worldview of drill and practice under which they were instructed. To be sure, instructive specialists have found that the instinctive convictions of educators about learning greatly affect their educational practices than hypothetical models got from research. Outside the institute, guardians and educational committees frequently don't figure out these new methodologies and may oppose their consolidation into their schools. At times, state schooling principles and educational program guides might go against new academic models recommended by research. At last, states and educational systems progressively require normalized finish of-grade tests as a feature of school responsibility, and instructors can see that as "instructing to the test" means quite a bit to their vocation accomplishment than contemplations of successful teaching method.

It isn't adequate for social researchers to exhibit the viability of new showing strategies and procedures, since instructive change expects regard for the array of social, social, and political powers that moderate the interpretation of hypothesis into training.

Perusing

Starting READING

Starting perusing includes obtaining of the numerous demonstrations, abilities, and information that empower people to fathom the importance of text. Perusing is a complex psycholinguistic movement and in this manner starting perusing is an extended and complex cycle by which the student secures mastery in the different perceptual, tangible, phonetic, mental, metacognitive, and interactive abilities that are engaged with proficient way of behaving. Through this interaction the kid acquires utilitarian information on the reasons, uses, and standards of the composing framework.

Encounters before Formal Reading Instruction

Albeit an enormous piece of education procurement happens inside the setting of formal understanding guidance, proficiency related mindfulness and information begin growing well before formal tutoring, through pre-understanding exercises and connections with print in the home and climate. The achievements before formal tutoring set up the kid for later school-related proficiency advancement.

There are significant contrasts among youngsters' initial proficiency encounters. A few youngsters are presented to a wide exhibit of early proficiency encounters. They are every now and again and routinely read to, they are presented to oral and composed language exercises, for example, playing on the PC or playing word games, they experience the practical utilization of print materials in their home and preschool conditions, and they have model grown-ups who worth perusing and use perusing in different deliberate ways. In 1990 Marilyn J. Adams assessed that kids from these standard homes are presented to a very long time of pre-perusing exercises before they enter 1st grade. Conversely, there are kids who are never or seldom read to, live in homes with not many books, are seldom presented to rich oral and composed language exercises, and communicate with not many grown-up models who use perusing and composing for their own motivations. These two gatherings of kids contrast broadly in their mindfulness and information on proficiency related ideas.

Ideas about print. Through rehashed associations with proficiency materials and exercises kids foster a consciousness of the nature and capability of text. Social schedules working on during one-on-one book perusing among guardians and youngsters work with kids' obtaining of ideas about print. From the beginning youngsters find out about how books are dealt with, the distinctions among pictures and print, the directionality of print, and the attributes of composed language-like schedules. Shared book perusing permits kids to foster a feeling of story structure where characters, the setting, and the plot make up the story. By noticing grown-ups' utilitarian utilization of education, youngsters likewise gain proficiency with the various motivations behind various proficiency exercises, for example, composing a basic food item list as opposed to composing a letter. In this way, when they are four years of age, kids likewise advance a considerable amount about the idea of print, including the names and hints of some letters, and will claim to "state" by writing as a feature of play exercises.

The procurement of the ideas about print is significant, and a few examinations have shown that such mindfulness predicts future understanding accomplishment and is corresponded with different proportions of understanding accomplishment. Accordingly, the improvement of ideas about print from the get-go in life appears to make the establishment whereupon more complex abilities are fabricated.

Language improvement. Communicated in language grows normally and easily inside the setting of social cooperation's locally. Except for the people who have a few actual difficulties all kids can deliver and grasp communicated in language normally right off the bat throughout everyday life. They show improvements in phonology, morphology, grammar, semantics, and jargon. Commitment to education exercises gives youngsters added chances to experience and explore different avenues regarding language. Book perusing, for example, offers different open doors for the kid to utilize language at a more dynamic and complex level than would be conceivable through communicated in language encounters. Youngsters learn to have a diminished dependence on prompt setting for correspondence. This decontextualized language is the language that they should depend on in most school exercises later on. Early education encounters likewise set the ground for development in meta-semantic abilities. Kids figure out how to ponder, play with, discuss, and break down language as well as utilizing it actually.

Phonological mindfulness. In sequential order composing frameworks depend on the portrayal of discourse sounds by letters. To comprehend the alphabetic guideline, youngsters should know that the expressed message can be separated into more modest units like words, syllables, and phonemes. Phonological mindfulness is the consciousness of and the capacity to control phonological portions like syllables, phonemes, and other intrasyllabic units, for example, beginning rimes in words. At the point when phonological mindfulness alludes to youngsters' aversion to the phonemes in words, it is called phonemic mindfulness.

Assignments in which kids are approached to separate, section, mix, or join phonological portions have been normally used to evaluate phonological mindfulness. Phonemic division and phonemic control errands yield areas of strength for especially of and connections with starting understanding obtaining. There are likewise concentrates on phonemic mindfulness that point out that there is a bidirectional connection between figuring out how to peruse and phonemic mindfulness.

While concentrates on kids' initial encounters with print meet on the end that these encounters and phonological mindfulness work with and set the ground for additional improvement in the securing of perusing, other exploration has researched the connection among IQ and understanding accomplishment. These examinations reason that IQ is simply pitifully connected with early understanding accomplishment.

Guidance in Reading

Kids are drenched in proper guidance in perusing once they enter kindergarten. Kids come to school with various degrees of mindfulness about print, and they experience in school new assumptions, new schedules, and new experiences that decisively widen their idea of proficiency. For kids whose language and proficiency encounters are nearer to those in the school setting, this change to school is generally simple.

Grasping the alphabetic rule. Before formal guidance in understanding starts, kids can as of now perceive specific words, particularly those happening regularly in their current circumstance, like Coca-Cola or McDonald's. All things considered, a recent report by Patricia E. Masonheimer and partners examining the elements to which kids take care of when they perceive these words showed that when the words were introduced without the logical signals, for example, logos, most youngsters as long as five years old neglected to recognize them accurately. Different examinations likewise propose that small kids perceive words in view of specific pieces of the printed word. Hence, before formal perusing guidance has started, most small kids can't get a handle on how the composing framework capabilities.

A sensational change happens when kids are presented to precise understanding guidance. Before they start to decipher autonomously, youngsters begin utilizing the phonetic upsides of letter names in recognizing words. Albeit this isn't yet inefficient word acknowledgment methodology, it is a major move toward utilizing the methodical connections that exist among discourse and the printed word. Full disentangling becomes conceivable when youngsters start to involve the full cluster of letters in words and guide them unto phonemes, accordingly exhibiting a comprehension of the alphabetic standard.

Efficiency and automaticity in word acknowledgment. It is absurd to expect to portray kids' perusing as useful except if they can perceive words that they have not experienced previously. As kids experience a developing number of letter designs during perusing, they bit by bit gather countless orthographic portrayals. Accordingly, rather than involving single letters for word acknowledgment they start depending on letter strings and their relating phonologies. This developing information on letter successions and spelling designs slowly permits peruses to handle words rapidly and without any problem.

Each time a peruse experiences a spelling design and takes care of the specific succession of letters in it, the example secures more strength and is thus recognized quicker and all the more productively during the following experience. On the off chance that then again as opposed to zeroing in on the whole succession, the pursuer's fixation is centered around settling a solitary letter, or on the other hand assuming one or a portion of the letters in the grouping can't be accurately recognized, the grouping may not be recognized as an element. As the youthful pursuer's information on the connections among spelling and sound develops, this information permits the kid to frame more grounded relationship among visual and phonological portrayals. Through experience with words on paper, particularly those of expanding intricacy, word acknowledgment turns into a programmed mental cycle, empowering the peruse to acquire expanding levels of familiarity. In this manner, contrasts in openness to print lead to contrasts in understanding expertise.

Perception. Perusing perception is a mind boggling expertise that requires a functioning cooperation between text components and the peruse. Since appreciation of text is a definitive objective in perusing, understanding cognizance processes is basic to the investigation of starting perusing.

Kids starting to peruse as of now have an advanced framework for oral language perception. Toward the finish of preschool most youngsters have advanced jargon and world information as well as morphological, semantic, and syntactic cycles that make oral language understanding conceivable.

There is significantly less exploration on understanding cycles in starting peruses, contrasted with concentrates on word handling. One of the reliable discoveries in cognizance research is that contrasted with more talented comprehends, untalented comprehends are additionally less gifted in unraveling. As a matter of fact, during the beginning phases of starting perusing, text cognizance is restricted to youngsters' expertise in translating. Until deciphering processes are fast and proficient, significant level appreciation processes are seriously restricted. There is presently uniting proof that for the two youngsters and grown-ups, troubles in understanding are connected with challenges in translating as well as to issues with working memory.

Other than being better at interpreting, gifted comprehends additionally have preferable worldwide language abilities over less talented comprehends. Studies have shown a causal connection among jargon and understanding. There is proof showing that jargon guidance prompts acquire in perception and improvement on semantic errands. It is likewise certain that both immediate and circuitous guidance in jargon lead to cognizance gains.

Gifted comprehends additionally have preferable meta-mental abilities over less talented comprehends. Talented comprehends know about how well they are grasping and utilize different perception techniques that guide them as they endeavor to figure out text.

Youthful peruses benefit from mental technique guidance. Guidance in mental techniques normally includes assisting understudies with monitoring their own mental cycles in perusing. Typically, an educator either models the utilization of perception methodologies or guides the understudies in the utilization of systems. Many ways to deal with mental system guidance permit peruses to rehearse their recently procured mental techniques with the instructor until the peruses ace their utilization.

To put it plainly, starting perusing guidance needs to zero in on youngsters' obtaining of letter-sound connections, as well as perception techniques to guarantee that both word acknowledgment and understanding abilities can grow at the same time.

Understanding

From 1997 to 2000 the National Reading Panel (NRP) completed a survey of examination based information about perusing and guidance, particularly in the early rudimentary grades. The exploration points applicable to early perusing and guidance that the NRP focused on were phonemic mindfulness guidance, phonics guidance, familiarity, jargon guidance, message understanding guidance, instructor planning, and perception techniques guidance.

The gathering that zeroed in on text perception guidance found in excess of 500 examinations on the educating of understanding guidance. Utilizing logical rules, for example, whether an investigation of a procedure guidance incorporated a benchmark group, they viewed that as a little more than 200 of these examinations were led adequately well to be sure that the ends in light of them are experimentally dependable.

Cognizance system guidance encourages dynamic perusing. The methodologies are intended to direct a peruse to turn out to be more mindful of one's self-understanding during perusing, to turn out to be more in charge of that comprehension, to make pictures connected with contents, to make realistic portrayals, to compose synopses, and to reply or to make up questions. Contingent upon what type it is, a system can be carried out previously, during, or after the reading of a text.

Gifted peruses might concoct procedures that help them comprehend and recollect what they read. Most perusers, nonetheless, don't unexpectedly imagine these systems. Except if they are unequivocally educated to apply mental systems they are not liable to learn, create, or use them. Perusers at all levels, truth be told, can profit from express understanding methodology guidance. An educator starts by showing or displaying a methodology. At times, the guidance is equal or conditional, implying that the educator initially carries out the methods and afterward the understudies slowly figure out how to execute them all alone. The cycle by which an understudy embraces the system an interaction that is classified "platform"- is much of the time a slow one. Perusers are first ready to experience the development of significance by a specialist peruse, the educator. As perusers figure out how to assume command over their own perusing by rehearsing and obtaining mental system methodology, they bit by bit incorporate the techniques and accomplish autonomous authority.

History of Comprehension Strategy Instruction

Interest in perusing cognizance systems started to develop as a piece of the new logical comprehension of perception that arose in the last many years of the 20th hundred years. In 1978 Walter Kitsch and Teen A. van Disk saw that a peruser is a functioning member with a text and that a peruser "understands" how thoughts in light of the text connect with each other by interpretive cooperation's between what the peruser gathers from the text and what the peruse definitely knows. They suggested that a peruser effectively fabricates significance as mental portrayals and stores them as semantic translations held in memory during perusing. These portrayals empower the memorable peruse and use what had been perused and perceived.

In a milestone 1979 review Ellen M. Marksman contemplated whether perusers would distinguish clear consistent inconsistencies in entries they read. She gave perusers a section about subterranean insects that demonstrated that when insects search away from their slope they transmit an undetectable compound with a smell that they use to view as their way home. The section additionally demonstrated, in any case, that insects have no nose and can't smell. Could perusers see that the section didn't check out? Could they perceive that they didn't grasp the section? How might they respond? Her upsetting finding was that youthful and mature perusers the same predominantly neglected to see either coherent or semantic irregularities in the texts. What guidance could assist perusers with being more aware of their comprehension and to learn procedures that could over-come these perception disappointments?

At about a similar time Dolores Durkin noticed perusing guidance in 4th grade homerooms throughout a school year. For the majority understudy perusers, 4th grade is a progress year from "figuring out how to peruse" to "perusing to learn." In a 1979 article Durkin revealed that there was next to no cognizance guidance in the study halls. Educators appointed questions and told understudies about content. In any case, in 75 hours of perusing guidance Durkin saw that year, educators gave just twenty minutes, under 1% of the time, to showing perusers how to grasp and advance new data from perusing. Her examinations and the others referred to above expected a serious interest in assisting understudies with gaining techniques to grasp and gain from perusing.

During the 1970s and mid 1980s examiners for the most part centered around training a singular technique to assist perusers with developing importance. There were in a real sense many investigations of individual perception systems. One model is Abby Adams and associates' 1982 examination applying the SQ3R (study, question, read, recount, and audit) strategy to 5th grade homerooms. SQ3R is a text pre-perusing realistic coordinator guidance created in 1941 for World War II military staff going through sped up courses. It is thought of as a "text reviewing" perception procedure guidance in that it guides perusers to search for the importance prior to perusing the text. In this guidance, perusers figure out how to utilize the text's headings, subheads, presentations, and rundowns to develop realistic schemata of the message content. As did a large number of the other perception procedure guidance specialists, Adams and her partners got positive results, finding that understudies with the pre-perusing guidance performed essentially higher on real short-answer tests than controlled bunch understudies.

By and large, many kinds of individual understanding system directions had all the earmarks of finding success in working on perusers' capacity to develop significance from text. With the noticed outcome of different individual procedure applications, there were a few surveys of this developing group of logical writing. In 1983 P. David Pearson and Margaret C. Gallagher arranged mental techniques by how instructors show the procedures, and Robert J. Tierney and James W. Cunningham's 1984 audit partitioned the mental systems into pre-perusing, during-perusing, and post-understanding exercises.

With the outcome of individual system guidance in further developing perusing cognizance measures recorded by research, center moved to utilizing blends of procedures to work with text understanding, principally in trial circumstances as opposed to in normal study halls. Among these was an extremely powerful 1984 investigation of "proportional instructing" of understanding by Annemarie S. Palincsar and Ann L. Brown. Proportional educating is a technique that in valves the slow arrival of obligation regarding completing a system to the perusers. It consolidates educator demonstrating and understudy practice on four mental techniques: expectation, explaining, summing up, and question age. Understudies who got this guidance showed stamped enhancement for various cognizance measures.

Progress of showing numerous procedures prompted the investigation of the viability of planning educators to show cognizance systems in normal, study hall settings. Two methodologies are imperative, to be specific Gerald G. Duffy and Laura R. Koehler's 1987 direct clarification model and Rachel Brown, Michael Pressley, and associates' 1996 conditional guidance approach. Direct clarification accentuates educator coordinated critical thinking, though value-based guidance, like corresponding instructing, utilizes educator coordinated activities with intelligent trades with understudies in homerooms. Both direct and value-based ways to deal with preparing instructors have delivered positive outcomes.

Techniques that Work

The NRP recognized twelve classes of appreciation guidance that have logical help for the end that they assist perusers with developing importance and in this way further develop understanding cognizance, remembering two classifications including the arrangement of educators for mental system guidance. These methodologies invigorate both sound and visual insight, enact memory and semantic handling, improve discernment, connect with syntactic information and handling, show account structure, and advance thinking. The procedures of undivided attention, cognizance checking, and earlier information utilize all advance tuning in and consciousness of one's reasoning or "internal discourse," a cycle underscored by the Russian clinician Lev Vygotsky during the 1920s. Mental symbolism, mental aide, and realistic coordinator guidance, then again, utilize perusers' visual creative mind and memory. Jargon guidance increments word and semantic information and critical thinking. Question addressing and address age require the entrance of what is known or perceived and the forecast of future occasions. Story construction and rundown guidance make consciousness of the association of thoughts and what is significant. At last, multiple strategy guidance joins the utilization of a few of these cycles together in adaptable and fitting ways. Research led in the last part of the 1990s likewise recommends that educators can figure out how to coordinate these sorts of procedure guidelines in homeroom settings and that friends working in agreeable learning circumstances can successfully coach each other in understanding methodologies.

Undivided attention. To train undivided attention, educators guide perusers in figuring out how to tune in while others read. The listening peruser follows the text as another understudy peruses out loud. The educator may likewise suggest conversation starters for the perusers to reply while they tune in. Undivided attention preparing further develops tuning in and understanding appreciation. It expands a pursuer's support in conversations, causes more smart reactions to questions, increments memory for the text, and concentrates and interest on material. For instance, in Gloria M. Boot's 1984 investigation of preparing basic listening systems with 4th grade to 6th grade medicinal perusers, there was a steady increment over the eighteen weeks of the concentrate in understudies' readiness to partake in bunch conversations and give more smart reactions to coordinate inquiries. In general, four investigations of this technique met NRP logical measures. The understudies in the undivided attention review went from 1st grade through 6th grade; they worked on in basic tuning in, basic perusing, and general understanding perception.

Appreciation checking. One can figure out how to pay attention to one's own perusing and to screen one's own appreciation. Guidance in cognizance monitoring during perusing assists perusers with dealing with their inward discourse as they read. Self-tuning in and self-checking of one's own comprehension during perusing advance more cautious perusing and better perception.

To show cognizance observing, an educator, while perusing out loud to a class, exhibits the methodology by intruding on her own perusing to "verbally process." She expresses to the class her own consciousness of challenges in figuring out words, expressions, provisos, or sentences in a message. At the point when a text presents potential understanding breakdowns, for example, new ideas or coherent irregularities in a section, the educator could think back in the message to attempt to take care of an issue, rehash the message content in additional recognizable terms, or forward search in the message to track down an answer. In the wake of noticing an educator model the perception observing technique, perusers are urged to complete similar strategies first with instructor framework and afterward all alone. Ultimately the understudy perusers assume a sense of ownership with perceiving perception hardships and for exhibiting ways of beating them (e.g., by speculating and thinking back or perusing forward in the text).

The educating of understanding checking is exceptionally powerful. The NRP found twenty investigations of understanding observing guidance with perusers in grades two through six that met logical rules. In them, perusers who were educated to self-screen understanding better one of the accompanying: their discovery of text irregularities, their memory for the text, or their presentation on normalized perusing appreciation tests.

Earlier information. Earlier information guidance is intended to help perusers in inferring their own insight that is applicable to grasping the text. An educator can enact earlier information by getting some information about points pertinent to the section, by showing the essential important information, by utilizing pre-perusing movement on related yet better-known subjects, by having the perusers foresee what will occur in the message in view of individual experience, by having perusers make relationship during perusing, and by seeing the story or message.

In fourteen examinations with understudies spreading over grades one through nine checked on by the NRP, earlier information guidance assisted perusers with enhancing review, being referred to replying, and in satisfied region and normalized reading comprehension execution. For instance, in a recent report, Teresa A. Roberts found that earlier information guidance emphatically affected both real and inferential appreciation execution with understudies in grades five and nine.

Mental symbolism. Mental symbolism guidance helps perusers to develop pictures that intently address the substance of what was perused and perceived. In 1986, subsequent to educating less-gifted 4th and 5th grade perusers in symbolism preparing, Linda B. Gambrel and Ruby J. Bundles had them perused stories with irregularities like those in the 1979 Marksman concentrate on referenced above and educated them "to make an image to you to help decide whether there is whatever isn't clear and straightforward about the story." Control understudies, that is to say, those without the symbolism preparing, were essentially approached to "give your best for help decide whether anything isn't clear and straightforward about the story." The outcomes were that symbolism prepared perusers were bound to distinguish irregularities than the controls. In four examinations with understudies in grades two through eight, the NRP found that psychological symbolism guidance prompted humble expansions in memory for the text that was imaged and improved peruser recognition of text irregularities.

Mental aides. Like mental symbolism guidance, mental aide guidance trains perusers to utilize an outside memory help, yet dissimilar to mental symbolism guidance, the memory helper picture can be one that doesn't be guaranteed to intently address the text. An educator exhibits how to build an image, catchphrase, or idea as an intermediary for an individual, idea, sentence, or entry, for example, utilizing a picture of a memorable "tailor" to remember the name "Taylor." These watchwords and pictures help later review. In five examinations analyzed by the NRP, mental aide guidance further developed peruser memory of the allocated watchwords and review for the sections read. For instance, in 1986 Ellen E. Peters and Joel R. Levin gave mental helper guidance to great and unfortunate perusers and afterward gave them entries about "renowned" individuals. When contrasted with the control subjects, the mental aide prepared understudies were bound to learn and recollect data about new ideas and individuals who were new to them.

Realistic coordinators. Realistic coordinator guidance tells perusers the best way to build shows that sort out one's thoughts in light of a perusing of the text.

Realistic coordinators target making familiarity with message designs, ideas and relations among ideas, and apparatuses to outwardly address message connections. They likewise help perusers recorded as a hard copy efficient outlines. Graphs, pictorial gadgets, and story guides can be generally used to frame the connections among text thoughts. This guidance is helpful for explanatory texts in happy regions like science or social examinations.

In eleven examinations checked on by the NRP that pre-owned realistic coordinators with perusers in grades four through eight, perusers by and large helped in recollecting what they read, in better understanding cognizance, or in superior accomplishment in friendly examinations or science courses. For instance, in 1991 Bonnie Armbruster and her partners looked at the viability of a realistic coordinator guidance that helped 4th and 5th grade sociology understudies to address the significant thoughts in a sociology text outwardly. Conversely, the control understudies' guidance comprised of exercise manual movement bearings suggested in the educator's version of the sociology course reading. The fifth-, yet not really the 4th grade understudies, who got the graphic coordinator mental methodology guidance scored higher on review and acknowledgment measures than the controls who got the exercise manual movement guidance.

Jargon guidance. There are many investigations on showing jargon yet hardly any on the connection between jargon guidance and cognizance. With regards to cognizance procedure guidance, jargon guidance advances new word meaning information by showing perusers semantic handling techniques. For instance, understudies figure out how to create inquiries concerning an obscure word by looking at how it connects with the text or seeing how a word changes importance relying upon the setting wherein it happens. The educator might show being a "word investigator," searching for relevant hints to see as a word's significance, examining words and word parts, and taking a gander at the encompassing text for pieces of information to a word's importance. For example, the word cognizance joins com, signifying "together" with pre-hens ion, signifying "ready to get a handle on in one's grasp." From this, a functional meaning of understanding can be built (e.g., assembling individual word implications to get a handle on a thought).

In three investigations of jargon guidance in a mental system setting with 4th grade understudies evaluated by the NRP, the guidance prompted progress in learning words, being used of word implications, and in expanded story understanding. For instance, in a recent report including fourth-graders getting jargon guidance, Isabel L. Beck and her associates trained the understudies to perform undertakings intended to require semantic handling. These understudies performed at a fundamentally more elevated level than pre-guidance matched controls on learning word implications, on handling educated jargon all the more effectively, and in undertakings more intelligent of cognizance. In the three NRP-audited studies, nonetheless, figuring out how to determine word implications didn't necessarily in all cases further develop normalized perception execution.

Question responding to. Question responding to centers the peruser around happy. By what means questions lead the understudy to zero in on causes and results. Question responding to guides understudies and persuades them to search in the text to track down replies. Guidance on question responding to prompts improvement in memory for what was perused, to improved addressing of inquiries subsequent to perusing, or to improvement in tracking down replies to inquiries in the text during perusing.

In a recent report, Taffy E. Raphael and Clyde A. Wonnacott prepared 4th grade and 6th grade perusers to break down questions, recognizing those questions that could be addressed by data in the section from questions that expected earlier information or data not in the text. The outcomes were that understudies who had gotten this guidance gave more excellent reactions to inquiries than a benchmark group of understudies. In seventeen examinations analyzed by the NRP for this technique, the outcomes were typically well defined for experimenter trial of inquiry responding to and were more prominent for lower-grade than for upper-grade perusers and more prominent with normal and less-gifted perusers than with successful perusers.

Question age. Educators show this system by creating questions so anyone might hear during perusing. Perusers then, at that point, work on creating questions and replies as they read the text. Educators give criticism on the nature of the inquiries posed or help the understudy in responding to the inquiry created. Educators train the understudies to assess whether their inquiries covered important data, whether questions connected with data gave in the text, and whether they, at the end of the day, could address the inquiries.

The logical proof that question age mental system guidance is powerful is areas of strength for exceptionally. In 1996 Barak Rosen shine and his partners led meta-examination of 26 inquiry age review with understudies from 3rd grade through school. Like individual exploratory examinations, a meta-investigation applies logical rules to get a quantitative evaluation of a guidance's viability. A meta-examination contrasts from single investigations, nonetheless, in that it gets a quantitative effect of a specific system by checking out at viability across a gathering of studies. Notwithstanding the Rosen shine meta-investigation, the NRP analyzed 27 inquiry age review with understudies from grades three through nine. Question age guidance during perusing helped perusing cognizance concerning further developed memory, in exactness in addressing questions, or in better mix and ID of fundamental thoughts. The proof that it further developed execution on normalized cognizance tests is blended.

Story structure. Story structure guidance is intended to assist perusers with grasping the who, what, where, when, and why of stories, what occurred, and what was finished and to construe causal connections between occasions. Readers learn to distinguish the fundamental characters of the story, where and when the story occurred, what the primary characters did, how the story finished, and how the principal characters felt. Perusers figure out how to develop a story map recording the setting, issue, objective, activity, and result of the story as they unfurl over the long haul.

Story structure guidance works on the capacity of perusers to respond to questions, to review what was perused, and to further develop standard perception test execution. The guidance likewise helps review, question responding to, and recognizing components of story structure. For instance, in 1983 Jill Fitzgerald and Daisy L. Spiegel found that guidance in account structure upgraded story structure information and meaningfully affected perusing perception with normal and sub optimal 4th grade understudies who had been distinguished as coming up short on a sharp feeling of story structure.

The NRP analyzed seventeen investigations utilizing story structure guidance with perusers going from 3rd grade through 6th grade. Story structure guidance worked on perusers' capacity to address short-answer questions and retell the story. In three of the examinations, state sanctioned tests were utilized for appraisal. Story structure guidance prompted better peruser scores in two of those reviews.

Rundown. Training perusers to sum up makes them more mindful of how thoughts in view of the text are connected. Perusers figure out how to distinguish fundamental thoughts, leave out subtleties, sum up, make point sentences, and eliminate overt repetitiveness. Through model and criticism, a peruser can be instructed to apply these outline rules to single-or numerous section entries by first summing up individual passages and afterward building a rundown or spatial association of the passage synopses.

In eighteen examinations on synopsis with understudies from grades three to eight analyzed by the NRP, perusers worked on the nature of their rundowns of text by recognizing the primary thoughts as well as by leaving out detail, including thoughts connected with the fundamental thought, summing up, and eliminating overt repetitiveness. Further, the guidance of rundown further develops memory for what is perused, both regarding free review and addressing questions. For instance, in 1984 Thomas W. Bean and Fern L. Steinway analyzed whether preparing 6th grade perusers in rules for synopsis created in 1983 by Ann L. Brown and Jeannie D. Day would further develop understanding. They found that perusers getting outline guidance either by rule-administered or instinctive summarization techniques performed better compared to controls who were told to track down primary thoughts however who had no unequivocal guidance. The summarization trained understudies essentially outflanked the benchmark group in the nature of their outlines and on a government sanctioned test.

Various technique guidance. Perusers can learn and deftly coordinate a few understanding techniques to develop significance from texts. Palincsar and Ann L. Earthy colored's proportional showing strategy, portrayed in 1984, educates perusers to utilize four principal systems during perusing: producing questions, summing up, looking for explanation, and anticipating what will happen later in the text. Extra methodologies may likewise be presented, including question responding to, making deductions, reaching determinations, tuning in, cognizance checking, verbally processing, and question expounding. The educator models procedures and, at times, makes sense of them as they are demonstrated. Then, at that point, the peruser, either alone or as a head of a gathering, applies the methodologies.

The proof shows that exhibition and rehashed utilization of the strategies leads to their advancing by perusers and improvement in understanding. In 1994 Rosen shine and Carla Meister led a meta-examination of sixteen equal showing review with understudies in grades one through eight. The vast majority of the perusers were above grade three. More vulnerable and more established perusers benefited most from complementary instructing. In eleven investigations of complementary showing in grades one through six assessed by the NRP however not covered by Rosen shine and Meister, proportional showing delivered clear certain enhancement for undertakings that include memory, summing up, and ID of principal thoughts.

Various system programs that don't utilize complementary educating chiefly have the understudy practice techniques with demonstrating or potentially criticism from the educator. In express, direct methodologies, the educator generally makes sense of a technique before the instructor models it during perusing.

Instructor groundwork for text perception guidance. Educators need to learn technique guidance to connect with understudies brilliantly and ideal spot during the perusing of a text. Educators likewise need to realize about mental cycles in perusing and how to show systems through clarification, exhibit, demonstrating, or intelligent procedures; how to permit perusers to learn and utilize individual methodologies; and how to show a methodology related to a few different techniques.

Four examinations directed in the last part of the 1980s and 1990s showed that educators who gain proficiency with various cognizance procedure guidance and use it in their homerooms further develop the perusing perception of their understudies, particularly the people who are sub optimal in expertise. Enhancements happened in topic learning and in execution on normalized perusing perception tests. In 1996 Rachel Brown, Michael Pressley, and partners trained educators to involve conditional procedure guidance in a yearlong program where understudies made perception gains. Exchange guidance includes teacher directed activities with intuitive trades with understudies in homerooms.

Helpful advancing by peers. Perusers might learn best when they are in friendly circumstances in which they are effectively drawn in with different students who are close to their equivalent degree of understanding. Helpful learning includes perusers perusing along with an accomplice or in little gatherings. As they read resoundingly and stand by listening to other people, the educator can direct them to involve any of the different systems for compelling understanding perception. At first the instructor might display perusing her exhibited utilization of a procedure. Then the understudy perusers do the showed exercises with an accomplice or in little understanding gatherings. Perusers alternate perusing and tuning in, seeking clarification on pressing issues, responding to questions, summing up, perceiving words, anticipating, and explaining. The perusers are urged to guide each other on procedures. Bunch agreeable guidance has been found to advance scholarly conversation, expanded understudy command over their learning, expanded social collaboration with friends, and reserve funds in educator time.

For instance, in 1998 Janette K. Klingender, Sharon Vaughn, and Jeanne S. Scum examined the viability of a helpful learning approach designed to energize socially and semantically different general instruction 4th grade understudies to utilize key perusing by utilizing different synopsis and explanation strategies during perusing. Understudies in the helpful learning classes made more prominent increases in understanding perception and equivalent increases in satisfied information than controls in measures that incorporated a normalized understanding test, a social examinations unit test, and audiotapes of gathering work.

In ten examinations on helpful learning of perception procedures checked on by the NRP, understudies effectively scholarly the understanding methodologies. Helpful learning can likewise be powerful for coordinating understudies with scholastic and actual incapacities into normal study halls. The social cooperation increments inspiration for learning and time spent by the students on assignments.

Suggestions for Future Research and Practice

Guidance of mental procedures for perusing perception has been fruitful across a wide number of review for perusers in grades three to eleven.

Regardless of these effective shows, there are numerous unanswered inquiries. Among these are whether sure methodologies are more proper than others for perusers of particular ages or various capacities, whether perception technique guidance would further develop execution and accomplishment in every substance region, whether effective guidance sums up across various kinds of texts, and whether understanding systems work better assuming what is being perused connects with the perusers' advantages. Scientists likewise need to figure out more about significant educator qualities that impact fruitful guidance of understanding appreciation, particularly as to dynamic cycles (e.g., knowing when to apply what system with which specific student[s]). At last, there has been little exploration that straightforwardly looks at changed techniques for educating perception. All the more should be known about "best methodologies" to perception guidance and the conditions under which they are fruitful. How can one best foster free perusers who have the capacities to comprehend what they read on their own?

Conclusion

Mental procedure guidance takes care of business to further develop perusers' perception execution. In her 2000 location to educators, Carol Minnick Santa, leader of the International Reading Association, noticed that "educating [comprehension] is much harder and more dynamic than showing phonemic mindfulness or language structures. Besides, viable cognizance guidance ... requests broad educator information." In 1993, following a five-year investigation of helping educators to execute perception system guidance, Gerald G. Duffy, a designer of the immediate guidance way to deal with mental methodology guidance, reasoned that training understudies to obtain and utilize systems requires a central "change in how instructor teachers and staff engineers work with educators and what they consider significant about figuring out how to be an instructor" (p. 244). Effective understanding instructors should be key themselves, organizing individual procedures and changing, changing, adjusting, testing, and moving strategies properly until perusers' perception issues are settled. For perusers to turn out to be great perusing planners requires instructors who have appreciation for reading systems.

CONTENT AREAS

Perusing in happy regions is likewise alluded to as topic perusing and disciplinary perusing and epitomizes what teachers call "perusing to learn." These terms allude to perusing, figuring out, learning, and utilizing content region, topic, or disciplinary texts like texts in science, history, or writing, to acquire, illustrating, and potentially making information in that discipline. Capability in perusing content region materials is impacted by: (1) the manners of people who read in the disciplines (counting such impacts as their degrees of foundation and technique information, how they might interpret the discipline, their perspectives and interest in the topic, and their capacity levels); (2) the objectives that understudies adjust for learning and how much those objectives are like the objectives that their educators have for their learning; (3) the design, trouble level, and tone of the texts; (4) the degree of understanding expected of the people (for instance, remembrance versus decisive reasoning); and (5) the structure where that understanding is shown, (for example, composed versus oral or review versus acknowledgment). In this way, perusing content region materials involves complex processes.

Teachers frequently express that "perusing to learn" is unique in relation to "figuring out how to peruse." When understudies figure out how to peruse, the emphasis is many times on the elocution and cognizance of account texts. Appreciation of these stories doesn't normally need aptitude in scholarly analysis and translation, in spite of the fact that educators look for strict, inferential, and evaluative/applied understandings. Perusing to learn, notwithstanding, centers around the comprehension and utilization of generally educational texts in disciplines like history and science and a blend of enlightening and scholarly texts in English. Perusing to learn requires disciplinary skill. While perusing a scholarly text, for instance, understudies benefit from knowing abstract pundits' thought process about and examine writing as a manual for their own translation and conversation of that text. While perusing a set of experiences text, understudies benefit from understanding the way that history specialists accumulate and decipher information and expound on verifiable occasions. Perusing to learn science requires an alternate arrangement of understandings than perusing to learn history, writing, or some other topic.

Level of foundation information, interest, objectives, and other understudy qualities have an effect in how well understudies can comprehend and involve the data in texts, yet happy region perusing experts differ about how much the way to deal with perusing contrasts relying on the discipline. Systems for understanding and applying what is perused will have a few commonalties across disciplines; by and large, in any case, the comprehension of disciplinary texts is inseparably attached to understandings of the discipline.

In a 1997 article Patricia Alexander placed that disciplinary skill is acquired as an element of three related impacts information, interest, and methodology use. That is, as one builds, the others do also. Alexander portrayed three degrees of disciplinary aptitude. At the degree of acclimation, information is disorderly, procedures are general, and interest is extraneous. At the degree of capability, information becomes coordinated, (for example, into processes in science), systems become more unambiguous, and interest turns out to be more characteristic. At the degree of capability, one might try and make information, techniques won't just be more unambiguous yet in addition become liquid and extremely productive, and interest will be intently attached to one's inward cravings. Understudies might move from acclimation to capability since they get snared on a subject and that snare assists them with turning out to be more inspired by different points, since they foster systems that assist them with learning all the more successfully, or in light of the fact that they might find out more and, hence, comprehend how better to involve techniques for learning. Regardless, information, interest, and methodology use are attached to the discipline instead of being viewed as broad builds.

Perusing in Three Disciplines: History, Science, and Literature

Disciplines vary in their strategies for making and showing information. Also, educators in the disciplines anticipate that understudies should figure out those distinctions and to involve them in gaining data from texts.

The instance of history. History texts are customarily composed as stories that are at times mixed with translation. For instance, an occasion, for example, the Tonkin Gulf episode of the Vietnam War might be portrayed successively, trailed by a section examining the significance of the occasion in deciding U.S. contribution in the conflict. Understudies frequently read verifiable texts as though they were "crates of realities" to be remembered in consecutive request, yet this methodology is credulous. Antiquarians, when requested to diversely peruse authentic texts, read them. In a 1992 article Samuel Wine burg detailed that students of history read verifiable texts as contentions. While perusing a few verifiable reports, they took part in obtaining (deciding the skill of the writer and the wellspring of the material), contextualization (deciding when it was composed and what encompassing impacts there may be), and validation (deciding if the texts concurred).

The distinctions in the manner understudies and history specialists read the archives can be ascribed to contrasts in disciplinary ability. That is, antiquarians know how authentic proof is gathered. They comprehend that there is the danger of predisposition in the choice course of that proof. They additionally realize that unique archives are some of the time challenging to decipher. The records are like bits of a riddle that should be collected without a previous boundary, with the last picture being a making of the history specialist. In deciphering those unique reports history specialists are impacted when period in which they live, the political and philosophical methodologies they have embraced, and previous verifiable translations, to give some examples impacts. What's more, students of history grasp the power relations that exist among antiquarians. They understand what considers great verifiable composition, model their own composition on that of others, and analyze the composition of their kindred students of history as needs be. History specialists grasp the components of their discipline and in this way perused verifiable texts with a basic eye.

In any case, the cycles of choosing and deciphering verifiable proof and expounding on authentic occasions is stowed away from the peruser of verifiable texts. In introducing history as a rational story, this data is darkened. Subsequently, it ultimately depends on educators of history to call to the consideration of understudies the components of the discipline that will assist them with participating in understanding history.

What are understudies expected to do when they read history texts? Commonly, understudies are supposed to participate in a few degrees of comprehension of history because of perusing verifiable texts. These incorporate a dominance of "current realities" of history. They incorporate figuring out consensual translations of history, like grasping different antiquarians' thoughts of the circumstances and end results of significant occasions. They likewise remember understudies' commitment for pondering these understandings for themselves. Understudies in history classes are frequently approached to make correlations and differences and to examine conceivable circumstances and logical results connections that poor person been made unequivocal in the texts. Understudies are additionally frequently expected to orchestrate data across a few texts. For example, they might be expected to peruse Benjamin Franklin's works and choose in what ways his thoughts had epitomized the standards of the Enlightenment. Here and there understudies are approached to check out at history according to alternate points of view. For example, they might be expected to peruse a few variants of an occasion to consider what the setting of those works meant for grasping about it. Understudies at times are approached to participate in the get-together of and translation of verifiable proof and to compose their understandings in report structure, for example, in a research project. At last, understudies are at times expected to take part in contemplating the philosophical parts of verifiable comprehension. For instance, they might be approached to consider whether notable individuals make imperative occasions or whether noteworthy events make notable individuals.

The custom in history classes for exhibiting these different understandings turns progressively toward article composing as understudies move from naiveté to ability and from lower-level dominance of authentic data to more elevated level decisive reasoning and translation. Hence, understudies need to have a complicated exhibit of methodologies for grasping verifiable texts and for showing that comprehension. These incorporate techniques for recollecting current realities of authentic occasions, participating in verifiable exploration, making correlations and differences, blending data across texts, composing expositions, and deliberate reflection about the idea of history and authentic composition. Though these procedures share normal components with methodologies required for different disciplines, they are, eventually, discipline explicit.

The instance of science. The hard sciences, for example, physical science and science lay on the suppositions of the logical technique. Researchers get it and utilize the logical technique as they continued looking for "truth." They stick to the rule of objectivity, understanding that their own predispositions and perceptual deficiencies might cause misinterpretations of proof. Consequently, they participate in trial and error utilizing controlled conditions whenever the situation allows and depend on mathematical as opposed to subjective appraisals of information as the primary determinants of logical standards. However, as researchers, they are as yet impacted by a few compelling components. The determination of examination subject, the utilization of specific estimation gadgets, the significance doled out to different logical discoveries, and the past understandings of the exploration point are instances of limitations that are to some extent socially and socially based. Which points get examined and which discoveries gain acknowledgment in mainstream researchers are elements of force relations among researchers, of need, and of the veracity of the discoveries. For instance, consider that it required many years for the thoughts of the seventeenth century Italian space expert and physicist Galileo

Galilei to be acknowledged by established researchers, or that cleansing methods were steadfastly opposed by established researchers notwithstanding proof that such strategies were fundamental.

Additionally, in science, data is consistently fractional and social. Since the functions of the regular world are darkened for people by the constraints of their perceptual and sociocultural understandings, logical understandings are dependably in a condition of transition. For instance, the thoughts regarding gravity and movement figured out by the English mathematician and physicist Isaac Newton (1642-1727) are useful on Earth however have become old fashioned in view of more current originations of quantum material science. Researchers figure out this motion; they have the disciplinary information important to assist them with basically perusing and assess logical texts. They likewise understand what considers composed confirmation of a logical finding. For instance, they realize that the revealing of a logical finding in the diary Science expects adherence to specific customary standards for logical detailing and has been namelessly explored (refereed) by a gathering of recognized researchers. They realize that such a report counts more than the bookkeeping of comparable discoveries in a neighborhood, no refereed distribution. Understudies, in any case, don't have the disciplinary information important to make these assessments. Capable perusing of science is to a limited extent subject to understudies acquiring that disciplinary information.

What are understudies expected to do as they read science texts? Normally, they are required to dominate an information base that addresses the ongoing understandings of mainstream researchers. These understandings include the recognizable proof of different components and their capability in completing normal cycles. For instance, understudies are expected to recognize the parts and figure out the activities of the human stomach related framework. They are additionally frequently expected to tackle issues or to make forecasts about processes in light of their logical understandings. For instance, an understudy who comprehends the way of a shot and the way things are determined may be approached to decide the time it would take a shot to arrive at the ground in the event that it was sent off at a specific speed at a specific direction from a specific level. At the end of the day, understudies should have the option to comprehend the jargon and ideas of what they read and apply that figuring out in new settings.

In attempting to comprehend the cycles of science, understudies might have to suspend their own thoughts for logical proof. In the investigation of gravity, for instance, understudies frequently have mistaken originations of how gravity functions in view of their natural yet deductively disproven suppositions. Understudies may believe that a heavier article will fall quicker than a lighter one, when, truly, weight or mass don't impact the speed of a shot as it tumbles to Earth. Researchers realize that weight has no impact since they have performed controlled tests. Understudies should suspend their natural convictions to become familiar with the logical data, and the people who comprehend the suppositions of the logical technique will more probable take part in that learning than understudies who don't.

Science texts are frequently viewed as hard to comprehend. Understudies grumble that ideas are not adequately expounded, the material expects a degree of foundation data that surpasses theirs, the jargon is excessively thick, and the substance is dull. Texts are significantly more diligently to comprehend when understudies start their perusing holding onto misinterpretations about the substance that disrupt their comprehension. Analysts have found that reputational text, or text that expressly portrays incorrect understandings and makes sense of why they are wrong, is more compelling at assisting understudies with learning irrational thoughts.

The instance of writing. Writing has its own disciplinary practices. Information on the way that scholarly specialists allude to such components as kind, portrayal, subject, struggle, imagery, and language use is significant. Furthermore, specialists in writing frequently participate in different sorts of understanding, for instance, putting a women's activist, Marxist, Freudian, or postmodern twist on the translation of a piece of writing. Specialists in writing comprehend the alternate points of view that are a vital part of the field. They comprehend that scholarly analysis has advanced over the long run; that the relationship of the writer, the text, and the peruser and their significance in understanding have changed; and that contentions rage over what is significant for understudies to peruse (the ordinance versus multicultural writing, for instance). Understudies might not have this disciplinary information however would benefit by it.

Understudies need to foster a typical language with which they can examine and expound on their understandings of text, and the practice in writing classes is for the showing of disciplinary skill to be in exposition structure. Also, they are frequently expected to apply their insight into the components of certain genres by taking part recorded as a hard copy scholarly texts themselves, like recorded as a hard copy verse or brief tales. What's more, they are some of the time expected to compose reports about creators or certain scholarly practices. The techniques for taking part in these exercises are very mind boggling, and, despite the fact that they require exacting, interpretive, and applied/evaluative reasoning, the manner by which this believing is utilized is unique in relation to how it is utilized in history and science.

The three disciplines-science, history, and writing are comparable in that all require thinking at exacting, inferential, and applied/evaluative levels. Likewise, perusing texts in these disciplines requires jargon information and key exertion. Yet, the disciplines are unique. For instance, science is all around organized, history less very much organized, and writing generally unstructured corresponding to what is settled upon as being "known."

Methodologies for Reading Content Area Texts

While examining methodology use, instructors find it valuable to make a differentiation between educator created and understudy produced systems. In both cases, however, content region experts squabble over whether general techniques can be utilized and applied across branches of knowledge or whether procedures should be discipline explicit. In actuality, most likely the two thoughts are valid.

An illustration of an educator coordinated system is list-bunch name. In this pre-understanding system, the educator requests and makes a rundown of all the data understudies definitely have some familiarity with the substance of what they are going to peruse. Then, at that point, she guides the understudies to bunch the things in the rundown into significant gatherings and to mark each significant gathering. From this action, the educator figures out what the understudies as of now comprehend and can, consequently, be more powerful in spanning any holes between data in the text and understudy information. Furthermore, the movement can be utilized to produce a rundown of inquiries that may be responded to by the text. These inquiries would then make perusing a more coordinated and intriguing action. The system can be applied across contents, however the rundowns that are produced and how the rundowns are utilized could vary relying on the discipline. For instance, in a set of experiences class, gatherings might incorporate occasions, strategies, and individuals. In science they might incorporate examples of conduct or cycles.

Concerning produced methodologies, to find lasting success in classes in any discipline, understudies should peruse determined to comprehend and contemplating the data at profound levels, sorting out the data into significant units, recollecting the data, and showing their insight in different ways.

Techniques, for example, reviewing, clarifying, and framing assist understudies with recognizing significant data to study; procedures, for example, outlining, planning, and idea cards assist understudies with arranging material across sources in significant ways; systems, for example, verbal practice assist understudies with recollecting and ponder the material; and methodologies, for example, anticipating and responding to test questions assist understudies with getting ready for showing their insight. Assuming understudies think at strict, inferential, and applied/evaluative levels, they will be bound to learn new data genuinely. However, despite the fact that these procedures can be applied across happy regions, they will, by and by, be different relying on the substance of the material. Proof that system use in one discipline can be moved to different disciplines without express guidance in technique adjustment is uncommon, thus it appears to be vital that understudies ought to get unequivocal procedure alteration guidance in each discipline.

All in all, the more discipline information they have, the more satisfied information they have, the more they are keen on the topic, the greater commonality they have with how information is made and organized in a specific discipline, and the more intently their objectives for learning match disciplinary objectives, the more probable it is that understudies will actually want to adjust general systems or make new ones to meet their discipline-explicit requirements for learning and applying the data in their substance region texts.

INTEREST

The strong facilitative impact of interest on scholarly execution overall has been deep rooted. With the end goal of this passage, the momentum conceptualization of interest is outlined, trailed by a survey of interest research on perusing.

The Conceptualization of Interest

Among the numerous conceptualizations of interest, the most widely recognized are to think about interest as a state or potentially as a demeanor. It has likewise been shown that interest has both mental and full of feeling (close to home) parts. Specialists likewise recognize individual and situational interest, with the previous focusing on private interest and the last option zeroing in on making fitting ecological settings.

Individual interest has been seen as a somewhat enduring inclination to reconnect with specific items and occasions. Expanded information, esteem, and positive influence have been associated with individual interest. Understudies bring to their scholastic experience an organization of individual interests, some like and some contradictory with study hall learning. Social classifications, for example, orientation and race additionally capability as individual interest factors that might influence study hall commitment.

Situational interest alludes to a mental state evoked by ecological improvements. The state is described by centered consideration and a prompt full of feeling response. The full of feeling part is by and large good, despite the fact that it might likewise incorporate a few pessimistic feelings. When set off, the response might possibly be kept up with. Situational wellsprings of interest in learning settings might be especially significant for teachers working with understudies who don't have performed individual interests in their school exercises.

In spite of the fact that distinctions exist among situational and individual interest, they are not dichotomous peculiarities. To begin with, both situational and individual interest incorporate an emotional part and finish in the mental condition of interest. Such a state is described by centered consideration, expanded mental working, and expanded and diligent movement. Second, agents yield that the two sorts of interest are content explicit and rise up out of the cooperation of the individual and viewpoints in the climate. Third, various specialists perceive that situational and individual interests might interface. Without a trace of the other, the job of individual or situational interest might be especially significant. For instance, individual interest in a subject might assist people with managing significant yet exhausting texts, while situational interest produced by texts might support inspiration in any event, when people have no specific interest in the point. What's more, situational interest might form over the long run into individual interest.

It has been found that point interest has both situational and individual parts. Point interest might play a particularly critical part in perusing and writing in schools since understudies normally need to manage text based on themes given by educators.

Interest and Reading Research

The main inquiries brought up in the writing on interest and perusing concerned the impact of interest on perusers' text handling and learning, the variables that add to perusers' advantage, and the particular cycles through which interest impacts learning. These issues are viewed as straightaway.

The impact of interest on perusers' text handling and learning. Up to the mid-1980s, the predominant view in instructive exploration was that capable perusers cycle and review text as per its progressive design. Hence it was accepted that perusers could review best the more significant thoughts at the more elevated levels of text structures. Since the mid-1980s, in any case, research has shown that perusers' all around shaped individual interests and their situational advantages (evoked by subjects and text portions) added to their understanding cognizance and learning. A few examinations have shown that expressly fascinating text portions and entries composed on exorbitant interest themes work with youngsters' as well as undergrads' perception, inferencing, and maintenance.

Analysts have likewise shown that interest influences the kind of discovering that happens. In particular, past expanding how much review, interest appears to considerably affect the nature of learning. Interest prompts more intricate and more profound handling of texts. In 2000 Mark McDaniel, Paula Waddell, Kraig Fins tad, and Tammy Bourg found that perusers drew in with tiresome accounts zeroed in on individual text components, for example, removing recommendation explicit substance, while perusers of fascinating texts would in general participate in authoritative handling of data. Moreover, their exploration recommends that text contrasting in interest might influence how much handling methodologies benefit memory execution.

Factors adding to perusers' advantage. Another significant instructive issue is to build how much fascinating perusing that understudies participate in.

The main part of the exploration in this space analyzed text qualities that add to making perusing materials seriously fascinating. In his fundamental 1979 paper, Roger Shank showed that specific ideas (e.g., passing, savagery, and sex) can be thought of "outright interests" that all around evoke people's advantage. In 1980 Walter Kitsch, alluding to these interests as "profound interests," recognized them from mental interests, which result from occasions that are engaged with complex mental designs or contain shock. Resulting research has recommended that an assortment of text qualities contribute in a positive manner to the intriguing quality and memorability of composed materials. Highlights that were viewed as wellsprings of situational interest incorporate curiosity, amazing data, power, visual symbolism, simplicity of perception, text union, and earlier information.

Message based interest can likewise be advanced by adjusting specific parts of the learning climate, for example, changing assignment introductions, curriculum materials, and people's self-guideline. For instance, in 1994 Gregg Schraw and R. S. Dennison had the option to change the intriguing quality and review of text materials by relegating for perusing different points of view on a similar subject. Furthermore, research has shown that introducing instructive materials in more significant, testing, as well as by and by important settings can animate interest. Changing the presence of others in the learning climate can likewise evoke interest. For instance, German analysts Lore Hoffman and P. Haussler showed the way that mono-instructive classes in material science can add to young ladies' expanded interest in the branch of knowledge. At long last, Carol Sansone and partners in a progression of studies demonstrated the way that people can self-manage to make errands really fascinating and in this manner to foster individual interest in exercises at first viewed as tiresome. Albeit these examinations didn't manage interest in perusing, they showed that interest in perusing could likewise be expanded by comparable techniques.

Explicit cycles through which interest impacts learning. Gregg Schraw and partners proposed in 1995 that interest ought to be considered a complex mental peculiarity impacted by different text and reader characteristic. A basic inquiry is the way the elicitation of interest prompts further developed review. One chance is that interest enacts text-handling techniques that outcome in perusers being participated in more profound level handling. Suzanne Wade and partners announced in 1999 that the associations perusers made among data and their earlier information or past experience expanded their advantage.

Mark Sadoski and partners recommended in 1993 that communicating however separate mental frameworks (verbal and nonverbal) can make sense of the connections among interest, understanding, and review. At the point when verbal materials are encoded through both of these frameworks, understanding and memory increment. The double coding proposed by Sadoski and partners appears to represent the impacts of a portion of the wellsprings of interest that have been viewed as related with expanded understanding and memory, like the handling of concrete, high-symbolism materials. In any case, some profoundly concrete and effectively possible data is more fascinating than other comparable data. Also, the enlightening meaning of power, oddity, shock, high private significance, and character distinguishing proof revealed in the writing to evoke interest don't appear to promote double encoding provoked by substantial language and mental symbolism. One more variable that has been related with interest, perusing, and expanded learning is consideration. Suzanne Hide contended that interest is related with programmed consideration that works with learning. All the more explicitly, she contended that such consideration liberates mental assets and prompts more effective handling and better review of data. In 2000 McDaniel, Waddill, Finstad, and Bourg announced experimental information supporting this position. At last, as interest without a doubt has areas of strength for a part, this viewpoint might assume a basic part in what interest means for realizing. The impact of feelings on premium, nonetheless, is yet to be completely examined in instructive examination.

Gaining FROM TEXT

Text permits individuals to discuss their thoughts with each other across existence. For sure, a huge piece of what every individual knows comes from understanding texts. Individuals who never find how to gain from text have solid requirements on what they can be aware and do. On cautious reflection, be that as it may, gaining from text is a more dubious theme than is promptly self-evident. Learning might be of greater when understudies experience the world straightforwardly as opposed to find out about it. Fourth graders who build electric circuits or twelfth graders who institute a fake preliminary might surely know more about the fundamental standards of power or the legal framework than if they had perused sections from their science or social examinations reading material. As engaging as advancing by doing may appear, it has its own limits. It is unreasonable to accept that understudies would have the option to get the comprehension of power that the nineteenth-century German physicist Georg Ohm had or the comprehension of the law that John Marshall, boss equity of the U.S. High Court from 1801 to 1835, had by rehashing similar school exercises even on many times. Through perusing, understudies can encounter the thinking of these specialists and come to know some of what they knew or know without finishing that very long periods of study or having equivalent measures of scholarly understanding. Fruitful learning relies upon a nearby match among peruser objectives, text qualities, peruser proficiencies, and informative setting.

Peruser Goals

Individuals read for some reasons. A secret sweetheart peruses another novel to be captivated and engaged. A cook peruses a recipe to effectively set up another dish. A guest peruses the phone directory to find a phone number. The secret sweetheart, cook, and guest will have associated the words, sentences, and passages of their messages together to be engaged, follow the arrangement of endorsed advances, or find the data they look for. All in all, they will have grasped effectively. In any case, they likely won't have learned a lot. The objective of the secret sweetheart is to be engaged, not to learn. While the cook and guest read to find data, this data most likely will stay in the text where it very well may be gotten to again when required as opposed to turn into a piece of every pursuer's information.

Perception, remembering, and learning require various cycles and various measures of exertion. Walter Kitsch, a mental therapist who has concentrated on text perception and learning, has demonstrated the way that youngsters can grasp, or review, a number-crunching issue without having the option to tackle it accurately and that grown-ups can review a bunch of headings without having the option to find particular area. To understand, perusers interface the different thoughts in a text into a sound entire that looks like the text. They know the implications of most words and can draw fundamental deductions between sentences, passages, and bigger segments of a message. As they draw these inductions, they recognize superordinate themes or thoughts from subtleties. Whenever requested to review a text not long after understanding it, they will generally recall the superordinate subjects, yet not the subtleties.

Remembering requires practice and consequently more exertion than perception. Perusers who re-read a text a few times, zeroing in consideration on the superordinate thoughts and a portion of the subtleties, will be better ready to imitate what they have practiced, especially whenever provoked. Remembrance is much of the time what understudies do when they study for a test. Assuming that the test has various decision or valid and misleading inquiries, remembrance can be a successful technique. Neither text cognizance nor retention alone, be that as it may, will bring about getting the hang of, as per Kitsch.

Kitsch observed that youngsters had the option to take care of an issue on the off chance that they could apply what they are familiar number-crunching and life overall to envision what is going on that addresses the subtleties in the issue. He recommended that learning happens when perusers can utilize their own important information to ponder, maybe rework, study, and hold or dispose of the substance in a text. Picture the expert culinary specialist following another recipe for a kind of dish that she has cooked ordinarily. As a result of her insight about fixings, planning decisions, cooking temperatures, and intensity sources, this culinary specialist would see any new elements, scrutinize the recipe, keep what she prefers, and add to what she definitely knows about setting up the dish. Learning achieves an adjustment of what perusers know, comprehend, and can do instead of basically what they recollect or grasp.

Texts for Learning

Gaining requires more from a text than fathom ability. Undoubtedly, understandability fills in as a watchman. Perusers who understand a text get an opportunity at gaining from it. The people who neglect to understand will advance little without significant mediation from the educator. Hundreds of years of grant on the features of viable composing joined by many years of understanding exploration have uncovered the qualities of intelligible text. Association is significant. Lucid texts are simpler to understand than ambiguous, ineffectively coordinated texts. In cognizant messages sentences and passages are coordinated around clear subtopics, and the general message follows a notable classification, like contention or clarification. On the off chance that the message has presentations, changes, ends, passage point sentences, and sign words that feature this association, perusers will fathom it better than they will a message without these elements. Notwithstanding association, perception is impacted by commonality and intriguing quality. Perusers understand texts better that are maximally educational, neither too recognizable nor excessively new, and that incorporate distinctive subtleties and guides to catch interest. However significant as text fathom ability may be, nonetheless, it doesn't address what understudies will gain from their perusing or whether they will learn anything by any stretch of the imagination.

What merits realizing? The logician Alfred North Whitehead found in tutoring the possibility to show significant understandings that understudies could use to get a handle on the turbulent stream of occasions that make up experience. In his 1974 book The Organization of Thought, he cautioned teachers, "Don't show an excessive number of subjects, [and] what you educate, instruct completely, holding onto on the couple of general thoughts which enlighten the entire, and relentlessly marshaling auxiliary realities round them" (Whitehead, p. 3.) The trouble, obviously, emerges in picking the couple of understandings to educate.

Ralph W. Tyler, in his exemplary 1949 book Basic Principles of Curriculum and Instruction, proposed five kinds of significant understandings. To begin with, subject experts accept that the significant understandings ought to come from the plan of the information spaces themselves. Second, moderates and kid clinicians keep up with that the objective of instruction is to deliver balanced grown-ups and that understudy needs ought to direct the selection of understandings. Third, sociologists, mindful of the necessities of society, contend that the understandings ought to be founded on anything the squeezing cultural issues are; the objective ofschooling is to deliver productive members of society. Fourth, instructive savants highlight significant essential life values as an aide, since they accept that the objective of training is to deliver a moral people. Fifth, instructive analysts make sense of that the understandings should be formatively proper; the objective of tutoring is to educate something. No educational program could successfully consolidate everything beneficial.

Subsequently, Tyler proposed that educational plan fashioners utilize their way of thinking of instruction and what they are familiar instructive brain science to choose which understandings to incorporate from understudy needs, society needs, and the space.

Other than being fathomable and introducing significant substance, particular kinds of texts are purposefully educational, planned explicitly to upgrade peruser learning. Contention and clarification, two recognizable classifications, are especially compelling informative text types. The two kinds marshal auxiliary realities around broad thoughts, the ideal educational methodology for showing significant understandings as per Whitehead. Contention offers realities and guides to help a case, or general proclamation. Twelfth graders considering the judiciary might read a message that presents insights concerning court choices to contend, "Through its choices, the Supreme Court impacts how the preliminaries in lower courts are directed." Explanation presents realities, models, delineations, and similarities requested consistently to direct a peruser from an ordinary comprehension toward the comprehension of a specialist. Fourth graders could peruse a clarification of power that presents the logical model of electric circuits. The clarification could start by portraying the ordinary experience of turning a light switch on and off. Next it could introduce the means for building a straightforward circuit and instances of circuits that light lights, houses, and whole towns. The clarification could show charts with bolts that show how power moves in every one of the circuits. It could finish up with a portrayal of the nuclear model and going with charts. Text highlights can significantly influence understudy learning.

Peruser Characteristics

To grasp a text, coordinate the thoughts in the text with what they definitely know and comprehend, and afterward build a model of the circumstance in the text, perusers should have the option to gain by a text's understandability and educational elements. Peruser information is vital. Perusers who are known about a text's point can depend on what they know to perceive significant thoughts and recognize them from subtleties. They can promptly distinguish the implications of recognizable words in the text and can utilize what they definitely know to deduce the implications of obscure words. Assuming they likewise realize normal message examples and how they are motioned in presentations, ends, changes, and point sentences, perusers can interface the different thoughts in the message into a rational entire that looks like the message. Information about contentions and clarifications might be especially significant. Perusers who hope to perceive and advance novel thoughts from perusing these two kinds will be definitely bound to get familiar with the thoughts than perusers who are negligent of them.

Yet, learning requires exceptional perusing methodologies past what perusers should be aware to have the option to grasp. In a 1997 article Susan R. Goldman, a mental clinician, checked on the broad work on learning procedures, including her very own portion work. She inferred that perusers who make sense of and elaborate what they are perusing and who have adaptable appreciation systems advance more from perusing than perusers who don't. The successful explainers effectively look for the sensible connections among the thoughts in a text. Pondering the connections helps effective students to remember related realities and models from their own insight. These procedures lead perusers to develop a model of the circumstance in the text firmly entwined with what they definitely know.

The Learning Context

Settings that really advance gaining from text put forth advancing as the objective for perusing, give understudies fathomable and "learnable" texts, draw associations between understudy information and perusing, and support and advance understudy pondering text. Understudies might peruse to finish jobs, to understand activities all the more completely, to instruct thoughts to each other, to sort out the significant thoughts in a text, and to plan reports, contentions, and clarifications. Every one of these learning objectives expects that perusers associate the thoughts in the texts to what they definitely know. Educators can advance associations by conceptualizing with the understudies, helping them to remember important encounters in and beyond class, empowering them to peruse from a few related texts, and matching perusing and experiential exercises. Advancing likewise expects perusers to look for the sensible connections among thoughts in a text. Settings that urge understudies to plan questions, sum up, make sense of, build realistic coordinators, and apply conventional composing designs help understudies to search out and distinguish the consistent association in a text. Since these systems require cognizant exertion, fruitful learning settings incorporate time for understudies to consider the associations that they are making, the coherent connections that they are recognizing, and whether they are effectively gaining from the text.

The very educational highlights that advance advancing overall will likewise uphold effective gaining from text. The message should be fathomable and present huge substance, in any case, and at any rate a portion of the guidance must focus on the thoughts introduced in the message. For fourth graders finding out about electric circuits or twelfth graders finding out about the legal framework, whether they gain from perusing text will rely upon the match among their objectives for perusing, the attributes of the text, their understanding methodologies, and the whole educational setting inside which their perusing happens.

Made in United States
Orlando, FL
01 October 2022